The Speech-Language Pathologist's Handbook for Inclusive School Practices

D0813501

The Speech-Language Pathologist's Handbook for Inclusive School Practices

by

Julie Causton, Ph.D.
Syracuse University

and

Chelsea P. Tracy-Bronson, M.A.
Syracuse University

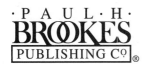

·P A U L·H·
BROOKES
PUBLISHING C⁰ ®

Baltimore • London • Sydney

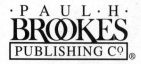

Paul H. Brookes Publishing Co.
Post Office Box 10624
Baltimore, Maryland 21285-0624
USA

www.brookespublishing.com

Typeset by Scribe, Inc., Philadelphia, Pennsylvania.
Manufactured in the United States of America by
Sheridan Books, Inc., Chelsea, Michigan.

Purchasers of *The Speech-Language Pathologist's Handbook for Inclusive School Practices* are granted permission to download, print, and/or photocopy the blank forms for educational purposes. None of the forms may be reproduced to generate revenue for any program or individual. *Unauthorized use beyond this privilege is prosecutable under federal law.* You will see the copyright protection notice at the bottom of each photocopiable form.

Individuals described in this book are composites or real people whose situations are masked and are based on the authors' experiences. In all instances, names and identifying details have been changed to protect confidentiality.

Cover image is ©iStockphoto.com/mcswin.

Photo of Julie Causton on page viii provided by Syracuse University.

The cartoons that appear at the beginning of each chapter are reprinted by permission from Giangreco, M.F. (2007). *Absurdities and realities of special education: The complete digital set* [CD]. Thousand Oaks, CA: Corwin Press.

Portions of this book were previously published in the following: *The Paraprofessional's Handbook for Effective Support in Inclusive Classrooms* by Julie Causton-Theoharis, Copyright © 2009 Paul H. Brookes Publishing Co., Inc. All rights reserved. *The Principal's Handbook for Leading Inclusive Schools* by Julie Causton & George Theoharis. Copyright © 2014 Paul H. Brookes Publishing Co., Inc. All rights reserved. *The Occupational Therapist's Handbook for Inclusive School Practices* by Julie Causton & Chelsea Tracy-Bronson. Copyright © 2014 Paul H. Brookes Publishing Co., Inc. All rights reserved.

Selected quotations in Chapters 2, 3, 5, and 6 are reprinted by permission from Giangreco, M.F. (1996). "The stairs didn't go anywhere!": A self-advocate's reflections on specialized services and their impact on people with disabilities. *Physical Disabilities: Education and Related Services, 14*(2), 1–12, as reprinted in Giangreco, M.F. (2004). "The stairs didn't go anywhere!": A self-advocate's reflections on specialized services and their impact on people with disabilities. In M. Nid, J. Rix, K. Sheehy, & K. Simmons (Eds.), *Inclusive education: diverse perspectives* (pp. 32–42). London: David Fulton Publishers in association with The Open University. Thousand Oaks, CA: Crown Press.

Library of Congress Cataloging-in-Publication Data

Causton, Julie.
   The speech-language pathologist's handbook for inclusive school practices / by Julie Causton, Ph.D., Syracuse University and Chelsea P. Tracy-Bronson, M.A., Syracuse University.
      pages   cm
   Includes bibliographical references and index.
   ISBN 978-1-59857-362-6 (pbk.)—ISBN 1-59857-362-4 (pbk.)—ISBN 978-1-59857-701-3 (EPUB)—
ISBN-10: 1-59857-701-8 (EPUB)
   1. Speech therapy—Handbooks, manuals, etc. 2. Inclusive education—Handbooks, manuals, etc. I. Tracy-Bronson, Chelsea P. II. Title.

   RC428.5.C38 2014
   616.85'506—dc23   2013027123

British Library Cataloguing in Publication data are available from the British Library.

2018   2017   2016   2015   2014

10   9   8   7   6   5   4   3   2   1

Contents

About the Forms

Purchasers of this book may download, print, and/or photocopy the blank forms for educational use. These materials are included with the print book and are also available at **www.brookespublishing.com/causton-slp** for both print and e-book buyers.

About the Authors

Julie Causton, Ph.D., is an expert in creating and maintaining inclusive schools. She is Associate Professor in the Inclusive and Special Education Program, Department of Teaching and Leadership, Syracuse University. She teaches courses on inclusion, differentiation, special education law, and collaboration. Her published works have appeared in such journals as *Behavioral Disorders, Equity & Excellence in Education, Exceptional Children, International Journal of Inclusive Education, Journal of Research in Childhood Education, Studies in Art Education,* and *TEACHING Exceptional Children.* Julie also works with families, schools, and districts directly to help to create truly inclusive schools.
She co-directs a summer leadership institute for school administrators focusing on issues of equity and inclusion as well as a school reform project called Schools of Promise. Her doctorate in special education is from the University of Wisconsin–Madison.

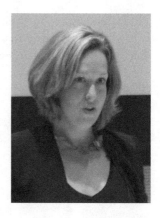

Chelsea P. Tracy-Bronson, M.A., is a former elementary educator who has focused her career on bringing inclusive educational opportunities to all. She is a graduate of Teachers College at Columbia University and is in the special education doctorate program at Syracuse University. She works with districts and schools to redesign services to create inclusive special education and related service provision. Her research and professional interests include inclusive school reform, special education leadership, curriculum design that allows access for all, differentiating instruction, educational technology, supporting students with significant disabilities in inclusive classrooms, and inclusive related service provision.

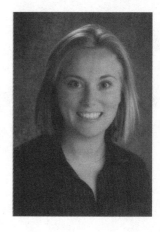

Foreword

I rejoiced when I was asked to write the foreword for this book! When presenting, I continually bring up the research and work of Julie Causton because it provides a foundational stronghold for many points I make about the importance of inclusive education, the idea and practice that everybody belongs and deserves to be educated with everyone else in their schools. I want to also acknowledge Chelsea P. Tracy-Bronson for her important work co-authoring this book because through her work she is changing lives. I am delighted because Julie, Chelsea, and I are kindred spirits in philosophy and practice.

One of the most important inclusive practice foundations of this book is exemplified through research conducted by Theoharis and Causton-Theoharis (2010). They examined the practice of pulling students out of the classroom to receive related services, including speech and language services, which is common in the United States. They found that the more significant the disability, the more likely the student was to be pulled out of the classroom to receive related services. The study concluded that this common practice is contrary to what students actually need considering their learning characteristics. Students with learning challenges need consistent, ongoing curriculum with units and lessons that are connected from day to day. Yet, what has happened in many schools is that students who need the most consistent, ongoing, connected curriculum in fact have the most fragmented schedules due to the pull-out model of related service delivery.

Some of you may ask, "I don't know another way, what can I do differently?" Let me give you an illustration of exciting, student-centered practices from my own experiences, which are expounded in this book.

Travis is a second-grade student who likes his tablet computer, his dog, pizza, and soccer. He has Down syndrome as an attribute. I have had the good fortune of being an inclusive classroom consultant for Travis since kindergarten, which I love because there is nothing better for me than witnessing someone learn and grow. During his school years, his team has refined their inclusive education practices in the areas of teaching and related professional services. Travis receives general education services, special education services, and related services in the general classroom environment.

His team has become savvy with the way they implement services. During one of my recent visits, I walked in during work time and here is what I found:

- Students were arranged in desk clusters of four to five students.

- There was quiet talking in the room.

- Students had the option of working alone in their desk area, working with another student or students in their desk area at a volume not above "2" (there is a voice chart of volume levels between 1 and 5, with "5" being the loudest), working alone on the floor, working on the floor with another student or students (with the same voice volume guideline applicable), or going to the library with a paraeducator.

- In addition to the desk clusters, there were four circular tables in the room. One table was for the general education teacher, Christina; one was for the special education teacher, Ryan; and the other two were for related services professionals (when I was in the room, one table was for speech and language [Tracy] and the other was for occupational therapy [Kim]). They all worked with students at a volume "2," consistently blending in with the volume in the rest of the classroom.

- When I entered the room, Travis was working with Tracy and another student. Tracy was using vocabulary words from the lesson the students just experienced for speech services. They were together for 15 minutes. When he was done, Travis went back to his desk cluster area. He looked around at the other students, who were working in their handwriting books. He looked at each student, took out his handwriting book, and started work. I wanted to jump up and applaud because Travis had a goal on his individualized education program to effectively initiate his work. He had made great gains since the previous year. Wonderful things had happened because he was modeling after his peers, who were great work models!

- Most significant, when talking with Travis, I found that his speech and language skills had noticeably improved to a new realm since the last time I had seen him. I was excited about the powerful peer models around him and about the way speech and language services were being implemented. Slam dunk!

- Teachers and related service professionals alike shared with me that they also worked with any student in the classroom based on current support needs in order to access and participate effectively in the lessons and assignments. Amen!

Many things delighted me about the observation. First, students had options and choices for how they did their work. Second, educators and related service professionals worked seamlessly with students on their caseload, in addition to those who had any educational support need. Third, the classroom environment seemed "just right," consisting of quiet voice volume with the option for any student to go to a quieter place, the library, if needed. Choice is good. Fourth, there seemed to be an astute understanding of the schedule and careful coordination to make sure everything in the classroom worked smoothly. I felt at home. More important, Travis felt at home!

Read this book carefully, using your common sense and your mind and heart. Carefully examine your practices. Are you promoting use of speech articulation, fluency, receptive language, expressive language, pragmatic language, oral motor skills, and so forth in the general school community? Are you providing services in real settings? This means general classrooms, hallways, the library, the cafeteria, the gym, and so forth. Have you embraced the idea that the purpose of speech and language services is to support the educational program and not to create separate services from the general classroom environment? Have you transcended your professional training and ditched the separate speech room in favor of *you* providing services everywhere with everyone else in the school where students really need to use skills?

If your answer to all these questions is "yes," thank you for being student centered, forward thinking, and progressive on behalf of proving excellent services to students. This book is for you because it will help you further refine your practices. If you answered "no" to any or all of these questions, this book is for you because you will develop progressive practices and see students gain speech and language skills to a degree you have never seen before!

Segregation of individuals with disabilities remains rampant in schools and in the world. I have written extensively about the extremely harmful practices of students with disabilities going to school on a separate bus, entering the school using a separate door, being educated in a separate wing of the school, being educated in a separate classroom, receiving related professional services in another separate room, sitting at a separate lunch table, and playing in separate, isolated areas of the playground (Schwarz, 2013). Carefully examine what is going on in your school. Are these practices any better than Rosa Parks sitting in a separate area of the bus?

In order for everyone to successfully live in the world together, we need to be educated together, receive support services together, play together, and live together. Otherwise, we are separating students from one another, taking away the ability for all students to learn from one another, and eliminating one of the most critical areas of learning—diversity education. In short, all kids need to learn daily about diversity in our schools and communities. There are generations of adults without disabilities in our world who did not grow up being educated in an inclusive environment. They have missed a very important part of their education and they show it by being indifferent to and/or pitying people with disabilities. When these adults were children, they experienced segregation in their day-to-day school careers. As a result, in adulthood, they believe that people with disabilities should live segregated in the community. Changing this practice must start in school.

Realize that by your own practices, you are central in abolishing segregation in your school. The fantastic news is this wonderful book will help you do just that! Get out your crystal ball and think about the future. Will the work you do impact the student when he or she becomes an adult in the general community? I have had the honor of working with many students during their school years and to continue to know them and work with them as adults. The good news is that I can honestly say that the more inclusive services are in school, the greater chance of successful "adult inclusion" in the community. You are a major part of the machine in making this happen.

Julie, Chelsea, and I need you to join us in redefining current speech and language practices in schools to effectively serve students in the most successful manner. When considering inclusive practice, speech and language is a very important learning area. It is an embedded skill and can strengthen every other educational area.

Read on and you will be changed in your thinking and practice. Be brave and do the right thing: All students deserve the best by receiving services that allow them to be equal members of their schools and community.

Hop on board—we are in this together on behalf of students! The more, the merrier, because you are an integral part of making schools become better.

Patrick Schwarz, Ph.D.
Professor, National Louis University
Chicago

REFERENCES

Schwarz, P. (2013). *From possibility to success: Achieving positive student outcomes in inclusive classrooms.* Portsmouth, NH: Heinemann.

Theoharis, G., & Causton-Theoharis, J. (2010). Include, belong, learn. *Educational Leadership, 68*(2): 35–38.

Preface

"Speech-language therapists are a unique balance of utilizing emotional engagement with the ability to utilize their education to create opportunities to offer everything necessary to help people who have the difficulty of processing and transferring thoughts to vocal engagement. It is of simple importance that they remember to not allow the language of 'impossible' or 'too many problems' to shut the door to the possibility of speech. With their support and the power of persistence, at age 12, I developed my voice and there are others I know that accomplished that at age 30 and older. To give life to a voice, they need often, courage to attend to the challenge with pleasure, and know they are needed and necessary to journey with us on the path to magnificent speech."

—Jamie Burke (Syracuse University student who has autism)

"I'M READY"

Tyler is a student who types to communicate. The speech-language pathologist (SLP), Moe, had been focusing on Tyler's initiation of conversation with peers during unstructured times throughout the school day. Moe also had been providing services in the classroom once per week to train Tyler's peers on having conversations with a nonverbal friend, showing them how to engage in written conversations, and facilitating social interactions. One particular week, Moe arranged lunch tables to facilitate social interaction based on interest. Each table had a discussion topic (e.g., LEGO building, music, Minecraft, sports). We think it is best to let Moe tell you the rest.

···········

Tyler is particularly fond of video games. I purposely added the Minecraft game as one of the discussion topics for a lunch table. This ensured that he was surrounded by other fourth-graders who were interested in similar hobbies. Before lunch, I took 10 minutes to have a class meeting during which I explained to students that the idea of the interest tables was to generate conversations with friends with similar hobbies. Students were so excited about this new lunch table arrangement and were especially eager to begin brainstorming lunch table topics to vote on for the following week. Once we arrived at the cafeteria, I facilitated peer interactions by initiating questions, then quickly fading support so students would talk to one another. I rotated around to all the tables, and kept a subtle and frequent eye on Tyler's table. Tyler and his classmates authentically discussed video-gaming techniques and the newest ways they discovered to pass the challenging levels. To be quite honest, I was lost in their conversation about characters, levels, and passwords. By the students' attentive listening, ability to pause when Tyler typed out his responses, and the continuation of conversation, it was clear that Tyler was an integral and valued member of this gaming discussion. Each Monday, students would vote on new table topics for lunch, and I would subtly be sure that there was at least one that would interest Tyler. After 3 weeks, I realized that this communication structuring technique worked so well to prompt Tyler to initiate and engage in real conversations with peers that I began working with other classrooms where students I provide services to are within, setting up a similar system.

One particular day, an aide responsible for watching students during lunch came running over to me. I was working in a different section of the cafeteria, facilitating discussions with a new class. "We've lost him. I can't find Tyler. He's not with his class anymore. I have no idea what happened!" In this moment, I quickly scanned the lunchroom, not seeing him anywhere. I ran to the office to let the secretary know. Within seconds I gasped upon hearing the following announcement read loud across the loud speakers, "Rainbow code. Rainbow code is now in effect. Mrs. Dool [the Principal], fourth-grade teachers, and all therapists please report to the office." We had lost Tyler.

After about 5 minutes, I spotted Tyler amidst a group of fourth-grade boys playing a game they made up called "Super Powers" on the playground. I asked a classmate standing toward the outside of the group, "Where have you been . . . and how long have you all been out here?" A classmate quickly responded, "We just came out to recess when Ms. Pea [a recess aide] said we could come out early if we were done eating our lunches. Well, Tyler typed on his tablet computer, 'I'm ready,' so we asked Ms. Pea if we could come out early, and we did. . . . We all came out and started playing. Why, what's the matter?" I was speechless for a moment. I chuckled to myself, smiled, and responded, "Absolutely nothing, nothing at all. Have fun with your friend!" Rainbow code was called off.

• • • • • • • • • •

What a difference communication makes in the lives of our students. In this case, authentic communication for Tyler led to natural friendships. Tyler's classmates heard him when he typed, "I'm ready." SLPs, like Moe, are invaluable members on instructional teams. She structured the lunch environment so that Tyler would have meaningful, unscripted conversations with classmates. It is the knowledge of language, pragmatics, augmentative and alternative communication, executive functioning and cognition, fluency, voice, resonance, and speech-sound production that make these professionals indispensable educational team members. Tyler's peers could hear that he was ready for more independence and interdependence. Let's hope we can hear the voices of our students as they become a much more integral part of inclusive environments.

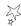

ON INCLUSION

Not a day goes by when we don't think about inclusion. When we both think of the amazing students we have had the privilege of teaching, we are reminded of what *teachers* they were to us. They have taught us that everyone has a right to belong, to have friends, to have engaging curricula, and to have powerful instruction. Everyone has a right to be treated with dignity and with gentle, respectful support; to be empowered to communicate and contribute; and to experience that learning is intimately connected with feeling like part of the classroom. Every student deserves to receive support in a warm and welcoming place. The more this happens, the more the school has created the environment for substantial learning. It isn't, therefore, just about creating a sense of belonging for belonging's sake; that sense of connection and welcome paves the way for self-affirming talk and friend-producing conversations, for academic and social growth. Therefore, this book is designed as a guide for SLPs and other team members as they work to include students with disabilities in gentle and respectful ways.

HOW THIS BOOK IS ORGANIZED

The first three chapters provide the context for the rest of the book: Chapter 1 explores the role of the SLP from multiple points of view, Chapter 2 provides background about special education, and Chapter 3 provides information about inclusive education. These first chapters provide the foundation necessary to more effectively interpret the rest of the book. Chapter 4 is designed to help SLPs rethink students. In Chapter 4, we will model looking at students through the lens of strengths and abilities for the sake of being able to reach and support all students more effectively. Chapters 5–8 are strategy-specific chapters that focus on collaboration, social supports, communication supports, academic supports, and behavioral supports. These strategy-specific chapters provide ideas that are immediately applicable in schools. The last chapter focuses on self-care and problem solving. The job of supporting those students in our school systems who pose the greatest challenges and require the most complex problem solving is not an easy one. Chapter 9 is meant to give helpful ideas for how SLPs can care for themselves in order to provide the best possible education for students. There are also numerous additional resources that SLPs will find particularly helpful.

WHO WILL FIND THIS BOOK USEFUL?

SLPs are one of the most critical factors to success because they are on the front lines, making daily decisions that support or impede access to curricula and peers. As more and more schools move toward inclusive education, we have heard from the SLPs we work with that their roles are changing; this book represents ideas and approaches we have used together that establish cutting-edge inclusive service provision. These SLPs who position themselves as critical to inclusion disrupt traditional thinking about therapy services provided in a pull-out setting. They demonstrate how SLPs are equally important partners in the work of doing inclusion well. SLPs need to be valued deeply because they play a key role in the facilitation of learning. Conversely, without appropriate training or support, they can disrupt the inclusion of students with disabilities by following the remove and remediate philosophy. Ultimately, a team approach to supporting students' communication in the classroom is necessary. Although this book will primarily serve SLPs who want to learn more about supporting students in inclusive classrooms, it is critical that these ideas be shared with the special educators, general educators, administrators, and parents who are team players in supporting students in inclusive school communities.

Practicing and preservice SLPs: This book is written specifically for practicing SLPs working in or hoping to work in inclusive classrooms in K–12 settings. However, this book is also perfect for students in SLP programs at colleges and universities; thus, we explain details that will be beneficial for individuals new to the field (i.e., practical strategies and suggestions, featured vignettes of practicing SLPs, individualized education programs, federal disability labels, and portions of the law).

Speech-language pathology assistants: This is an excellent book to read along with a speech-language pathology assistant. It can then be used to discuss key ideas and practices they are responsible for carrying out under appropriate supervision.

Special educators: Special educators support students in inclusive classrooms. This book identifies approaches, strategies, and suggestions for supporting all students in inclusive classrooms. This book can be used for SLPs and special educators to read and discuss together in a professional development or book club format.

General educators: General educators are an important part of the classroom team. Learning more about SLPs and support strategies allows general educators to offer a seamless and thoughtful integration of services.

Administrators: This book is an invaluable resource for principals to use as a resource along with SLPs who seek to build schoolwide inclusive practices.

Parents of students with special needs: Parents can benefit from this book by understanding inclusive models of speech and language services that lead to increased commitment from the entire educational team for authentic, meaningful communication throughout the school day rather than focusing simply on "speech time." For them, this book can be a resource to secure the appropriate training and support for the SLP working with their child.

Professional development personnel: This book offers cutting-edge approaches and resources for providing therapy to students with disabilities that are useful for any speech-language pathology training or team training.

This book is a companion guide to *The Paraprofessional's Handbook for Effective Support in Inclusive Classrooms* (Paul H. Brookes Publishing Co., 2009), *The Principal's Handbook for Leading Inclusive Schools* (Paul H. Brookes Publishing Co., 2014), and *The Occupational Therapist's Handbook for Inclusive School Practices* (Paul H. Brookes Publishing Co., 2014) so that educational teams can gain shared knowledge. It is purposefully organized in the same way, using the same headings and much of the same information, shared from the SLP's perspective and point of view. We are currently in the process of writing more handbooks and hope to see all of these books used together as teams work collaboratively to support all students in inclusive settings.

Acknowledgments

JULIE'S ACKNOWLEDGMENTS

This book is about support—meaningful, thoughtful, humanistic support—that allows people to reach their full potential, become their best selves, and do their best work. Support is not only for those we deem in need of support; it is a human need that is essential for everyone. Support isn't just for those we think of as "different" or "special." This work is a call for a different paradigm in schools—where support is available for all to create a community essential for learning.

Indeed, this book and my own academic career would not have been possible without all sorts of support that give me confidence—in schools and college class-rooms, on academic panels, and in school district in-services. Therefore, I feel it is necessary to thank the sizeable community of students, teachers, scholars, family, and friends who have supported me in both visible and invisible ways as we have written this book. This journey is driven by a vision of substantive and meaningful inclusion for all children. I want to thank the many individuals who have helped me see the importance of the journey, imagine the route, and stay the course.

To my students: I have worked with many students over the years, and each taught me something new. I would especially like to thank those who have forced me to think in new ways: Chelsea, Joryann, Ricki, Josh, Moua, Brett, Shawnee, Adam, Trevor, and Gabe.

To my teaching partner: Kathie Crandall, my friend, you taught me that laughter is truly the best indicator of learning.

To my teachers: Lou Brown, your belief in inclusion has inspired me throughout my entire academic career, and Alice Udvari-Solner, you have sustained me with your intellectual vision, creativity, and commitment to *all* children. Your work has touched every aspect of this book, and it is impossible to say where your influence ends. I also thank Kimber Malmgren and Colleen Capper, whose mentorship has made my career in education possible.

To my friends and colleagues: To George Theoharis, the best co-parent anyone could ask for, a daily sounding board, co-author, and dear friend. Chelsea Tracy-Bronson,

Sharon Dotger, Paula Kluth, Michael Giangreco, Doug Biklen, Christi Kasa, Corrine Roth Smith, Beth Ferri, Thomas Bull, Corrie Burdick, Meghan Cosier, Christy Ashby, Tara Affolter, and Steve Hoffman: You help me through each and every day and remind me that there is much more to life than work.

To Brookes Publishing Co.: I thank Rebecca Lazo, Steve Plocher, and all of the Brookes staff for your helpful suggestions and creative vision.

To Stephanie Perotti: You make me laugh every day and bring an enthusiasm and an energy to my life that is unparalleled. Thank you!

To my family: I thank Ella Theoharis and Sam Theoharis. You fill me with joy, your creativity inspires me, and you remind me of the importance of this work every single day. Thanks to Gail Andre, Jeff Causton, and Kristine Causton, for being excited about the importance of my work.

CHELSEA'S ACKNOWLEDGMENTS

I have the deepest gratitude for the individuals in my personal, teaching, and academic spheres who have shared this journey with me. The work in this book grows out of the experiences I have had throughout my career that have spanned the many aspects of schooling and are sprinkled throughout the chapters.

To my students: I wish to acknowledge my first students who helped me conceptualize inclusive education. Quin taught me that the best teachers are compassionate and deeply embedded into the lives of our students. Michael convinced me that facilitating social interdependence is gift that does not stop giving. I am also especially grateful to James, Tyler, Neleah, Camryn, Shantell, Maylee, Aaliyah, Emma, Hunter, Adam, Ella, Evan, and Mikayla, who taught me to think and teach in different ways, create exciting learning experiences, and to be passionate about teaching.

To my colleagues: Thanks to Katie, who is the epitome of an inclusive teacher. Beth, Maria, and Lauren, with whom I worked alongside during my initial teaching experiences: thank you for facilitating my passion to ensure access to meaningful curriculum for all learners. Along with co-planning and co-instructing, Lisa, my teaching partner, showed me how to dance the dance and make learning fun! Jenn taught me that life is washable and the best learning is messy. Thanks to Carolyn, the Tigger of the school, and to Diane, Kelly, Erin, and Amy, who all taught me their tricks of the art of teaching.

To my teachers: Several mentors have shaped my thinking about inclusive education and designing accessible curriculum. I am grateful to Julie Causton, whose work touches on so many aspects of every lesson I have taught and whose work has been the inspiring force behind so much of what I have accomplished. Thomas Hatch's work in school change shaped my teaching and helped me create a vision for the future. George Theoharis always demonstrated that a compassionate disposition and a focus on all students are key ingredients for any leadership recipe. It was Karen Zumwalt's teaching, vision, and mentoring that pushed me to be an academic scholar. Thanks also to Christy Ashby, who stressed the importance of access and communication for students with significant disabilities that empowered me to create meaningful relationships with individuals who are nonverbal. And a special thank you is extended to many excellent Syracuse University and Teachers College, Columbia University, professors.

To my friends and family: Aaryn, Elise, Shelby, Brian, Fred, Vicky, Ian, Vicky, Eric, and Constance remind me of the importance of family and friendship. Heith and Holly, you are two of the most fun, loving, and caring souls in my life, whose endless support I cherish. Inga, you are a best friend who balances me daily. J.R., you are my rock, my best friend, and my Zuppa; I am thankful for all the adventures that fill our lives. For my parents, thank you for making my dreams become reality. Your love, interest, and passion in the work that I do matters.

*To all of the amazing students who have touched our lives
and to Ella and Sam, the greatest teachers*

1

The Speech-Language Pathologist

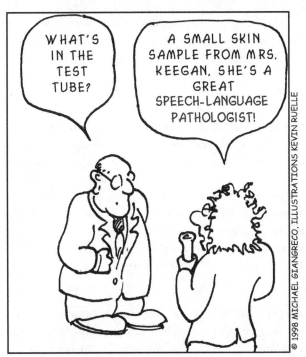

DESPITE THE BIO-ETHICAL CONTROVERSIES
MAGGIE FAVORS HUMAN CLONING.

"Changing from predominately pulling students out to inclusive service has been an exciting challenge of creativity. I have really enjoyed the process of discovering new ways to support students. . . . I think teaching students in the context of peers and rich communication has made my services more effective."

—Erin (speech-language pathologist)

Like Erin, many speech-language pathologists (SLPs) are navigating new methods to deliver their related services within inclusive classrooms in order to ensure that students with disabilities have continued access to quality instruction and related services throughout the course of the school day without the disruption of pull-out sessions. SLPs across the country envision different service provision models aimed to support students with disabilities. Whether you are a preservice SLP or someone who has been practicing in the field for years, this book is designed to help you take on the role of providing inclusive services with ease. Some of the information in Chapters 1 and 2 may be a review for those who are seasoned SLPs; feel free to skim those sections if they are familiar to you already. Our goal is that this book provides you with useful ideas to create more inclusive service provision. This book is meant to provide essential knowledge and guidance about 1) what it means to be an SLP, 2) special education basics, 3) inclusive education, 4) how to work within a collaborative team, 5) new ways to think about the students to whom you provide services, 6) how to provide social supports, 7) implementing therapy provision that aligns with academic goals, 8) behavioral supports, and 9) how to take care of yourself while doing this important work.

· · · · · · · · · ·

In one inclusive second-grade classroom the SLP and teacher sit down with the specific communication goals of the two students who receive speech-language services in that classroom. They plan an upcoming English/language arts lesson that not only meets the needs of all the students but have embedded individualized education program (IEP) goals right within the lesson. So, as the lesson is carried out, the SLP teacher has a center, the general education teacher has a center, and the special educator has a center. All the students rotate through all of the centers and at each center the individual goals are embedded and practiced with each adult running the center. Data are collected on each of the goals, and they plan again next week.

· · · · · · · · · ·

The SLP was vital in embedding communication and speech skills not only for the two students who received speech services, but also for the entire class. Furthermore, the two students who need intensive speech support were able to receive these services without a disruption to their typical classroom routine and without missing general education content. This example highlights possible contributions a school-based SLP can make on an educational team to deliver instruction to all students. This chapter will familiarize you with the evolving job of the school-based SLP. We will outline the history of SLPs, the definition of speech and language therapy, the roles of the SLP, the benefits of SLPs, the different types of settings in which school-based SLPs work, the most common professional responsibilities for SLPs, and some commonly asked questions.

THE HISTORY OF SPEECH-LANGUAGE PATHOLOGISTS

The history of inclusive education has had a large impact on the role of school-based SLPs. It has only been since the passage of the Education for All Handicapped Children Act of 1975 (PL 94-142) that students with disabilities have had a legally protected right to attend public school. Prior to that, students with disabilities were educated mainly in the home, in segregated settings, or in institutions. In the 1950s and 1960s, children with disabilities were in segregated educational and rehabilitative programs. As a result, therapists primarily worked in these separate settings only for children who required their services. In the 1970s and 1980s, however, a strong, parent-driven push began for including children with disabilities in general education settings alongside students without disabilities. At this time, the inclusive education initiative began (Will, 1986), and parents began to learn about the idea of *mainstreaming* or *inclusion*. The role of SLPs shifted accordingly, as students with disabilities began participating in general education classrooms.

By the 1990s, a wider array of students with more significant disabilities was included in classrooms across all grade levels in school. From 2000 to the present, inclusive education has been a legal mandate. The No Child Left Behind Act (NCLB) of 2001 (PL 107-110) initially set accountability and educational standards for all children, including students with disabilities. The federal legislation that had particular impact on students with disabilities was the reauthorization of the Individuals with Disabilities Education Improvement Act (IDEA) of 2004 (PL 108-446), which established outcome expectations for students with disabilities receiving special education and related services. In the Findings section of IDEA 2004, Congress acknowledged that the purpose was to "ensure that all children with disabilities have available . . . a free appropriate public education that emphasizes special education and related services designed to meet their unique needs . . ." (20 U.S.C. 1400 [c]). Therefore, students with disabilities were entitled to receive related services. That is, under federal legislation, the role of SLPs is to "assist a child with a disability to benefit from special education" (IDEA, 2004, 20 U.S.C. §602 [26][A]) and to ensure these students have "access to the general education curriculum in the regular classroom, to the maximum extent possible" (IDEA, 2004, 20 U.S.C. §601[c][5][A]). As educational policy and practice have evolved and more students with significant disabilities are being included in general education settings, it is clear that SLPs who work primarily with children work under the provisions of IDEA, and their services now take place in schools (Swinth, Spencer, & Leslie, 2007). Presently, "more than 57% of certified speech-language pathologists work in educational facilities" (American Speech-Language-Hearing Association [ASHA], 2013). Furthermore, "it is essential that speech-language pathologists' roles and responsibilities be redefined in light of substantive changes that have taken place in schools, as well as in the discipline of speech-language pathology" (ASHA, 2010). As mentioned, our intention is that this book be a practical resource for information and strategies for school-based SLPs who take on the role of providing services within inclusive contexts. Thus, we now consider what the job of SLP means in educational settings.

WHAT DOES *SPEECH-LANGUAGE PATHOLOGIST* MEAN?

You already have a vast understanding about school-based SLPs. Here we complement this knowledge by reviewing what federal legislation describes. SLPs within education settings are integral members of the educational team, providing students with disabilities access to communication and language supports. The job of the SLP is described in section 300.34 of IDEA 2004 as a related service. "Related services means . . . supportive services as are required to assist a child with a disability to benefit from special education" (20 U.S.C. § 300.34). Specifically, the definition of speech and language therapy is in section 15 of IDEA 2004:

> Speech-language pathology services includes: (a) identification of children with speech or language impairments; (b) diagnosis and appraisal of specific speech or language impairments; (c) referral for medical or other professional attention necessary for the habilitation of speech and language impairments; provision of speech and language services for the habilitation or prevention of communicative impairments; and, (d) counseling and guidance of parents, children, and teachers regarding speech and language impairments. (20 U.S.C. § 300.34 [c][15])

In other words, SLPs are qualified professionals who identify and diagnose speech and language impairments as well as provide services to improve communicative functioning to allow a student with a disability to benefit from special education services.

NCLB 2001 considers SLPs as pupil services personnel in section 9101.36:

> The term pupil services personnel means . . . other qualified professional personnel involved in providing assessment, diagnosis, counseling, educational, therapeutic, and other necessary services as part of a comprehensive program to meet student needs. (section 9101, paragraph 36)

We have provided the legal definition of SLP (IDEA, 2004) and pupil services (NCLB, 2001); now, we will discuss what this means in practical terms and what it actually looks like in the classroom.

SPEECH-LANGUAGE PATHOLOGIST: FROM PULL-OUT AND CASELOAD TO INCLUSIVE, COLLABORATIVE WORKLOADS

The role of SLP is essential in public schools today. SLPs are faced with growing caseloads, and we must be sure these are reasonable. ASHA (2010) argued, "For SLPs to be productive in the many roles and responsibilities for which their expertise prepares them, they must have reasonable workloads . . . new or expanded roles cannot merely be additions to an already full workload." This increase in caseload is attributable to many factors. The number has increased primarily because many more students with significant disabilities (e.g., autism spectrum disorders, cognitive disabilities) are included in general education classrooms. In addition, there has been a slow increase in the number of students who are being identified as having disabilities. Many educators view the consultation and classroom-based support of an SLP as key for students with disabilities to benefit from special education in the context of general education classrooms.

Consequently, the role of SLP has become more complex as it moved from a direct, hands-on, pull-out only service model to classroom-based therapist. In the past, students with significant disabilities were routinely educated within segregated classrooms with a focus on functional and behavioral skills. Educational goals for these students were essentially limited to life skills and job-related tasks. As a result, the role of SLPs was mainly to support these life skills in relation to language and communication and was performed through segregated environments. ASHA (1996) stated,

> Traditionally, service delivery was based on a medical model in which the clinical process was often separated into diagnostic and treatment functions that encouraged isolated, individualized assessment and treatment. Frequently, when clinical speech-language pathology services were rendered, there was insufficient communication between the speech-language pathologist and other instruction staff.

Now, educators in the field have learned that students with disabilities are just as capable of learning as their general education counterparts. Consequently, the goals many students now have in their individualized education programs (IEPs) closely resemble those of their same-age peers. Under federal law, therapists are required to provide related service supports and work in conjunction with educators to ensure that students with significant disabilities can function adequately in general education classrooms in order to benefit from special education (IDEA, 2004) and provide these therapeutic services as a "comprehensive program to meet student needs" (NCLB, 2001). ASHA also adheres to the notion of collaborative partnerships to meet students' needs and remain in compliance with federal and state mandates (ASHA, 2010).

Another shift that some SLPs have seen is from thinking about caseload numbers toward comprehensive workload (Schraeder, 2013). This workload takes into account the work activities that therapists provide to benefit students, including consultation, innovative methods to provide direct services in general education environments, meetings with educational teams, data collection, and evaluations (ASHA, 2002a). As stated by ASHA,

> School systems and SLPs themselves must make ethical and judicious decisions, consistent with legal mandates, about the services they provide. They must balance their scope of work to use their expertise most effectively and efficiently. New or expanded roles cannot merely be additions to an already full workload.

Based on federal legislation and the aforementioned national public schooling trends, SLPs have become integral team members with increasingly challenging responsibilities to provide services to students in their least restrictive environment (LRE).

THE ROLE OF SPEECH-LANGUAGE PATHOLOGISTS TODAY

School-based SLPs have varied responsibilities. Your role is likely determined by the needs of students who receive therapy services and the unique school context. ASHA (2010) outlined the professional contributions SLPs bring to schools in order to "promote efficient and effective outcomes for students." SLPs have professional responsibilities that include a range of focus areas. Table 1.1 describes typical responsibilities of SLPs and includes examples of supports that can be provided for students within the LRE. To be clear, these are types of professional responsibilities you may have as an SLP, but your role may change based on the needs of your students and the unique educational context.

BENEFITS OF SPEECH-LANGUAGE PATHOLOGISTS

SLPs provide related services to children. Additional benefits include collaborating with educators, other related service providers, administrators, and families to support the IEP goals of students with disabilities within the educational environment of school. As a related service, speech-language pathology serves a significant supportive role in enabling the student with a disability to participate in and benefit from special education. In fact, federal legislation requires that a free appropriate public education (FAPE) that includes special education and related services be "provided in conformity with the individualized education program" (IDEA, 2004, 20 U.S.C. 1401[9]). As such, the speech-language pathology service provision occurs in the school context where the need occurs. For many students with disabilities, their IEPs are now delivered fully within general education classrooms.

IN WHAT SETTINGS MIGHT I WORK?

Although this book focuses on supporting students in inclusive classrooms, you might find yourself in different types of classrooms. Brief definitions of the various settings in which you may find yourself follow.

Inclusive Classrooms

Inclusive classrooms are educational environments in which students with and without disabilities are educated together. The needs, supports, and therapy of all learners are addressed in inclusive, heterogeneous environments. Other terms you might hear are *general education classroom, third-grade classroom,* or *typical classroom.* A more outdated term for an inclusive classroom is a *mainstreamed classroom.* Therapy interventions and supports can be delivered right within inclusive classrooms. More information about inclusive education can be found in Chapter 3.

Table 1.1. Typical responsibilities of speech-language pathologists

Focus area	Examples of professional responsibilities
Speech sound production	Facilitating small-group cooperative games that focus on certain phonological sounds (e.g., /s/ and /z/, /sh/ and /ch/) Leading songs, word chants, or poems that focus on target sounds in the classroom Picking guided reading books for target students that focus on specific sounds Suggesting transition strategies that involve repeated phrases (e.g., "clean up, clean up, everybody do their job") Collaborating with the music teacher to sing songs that repeat troublesome consonant clusters
Voice	Planning a station activity during reading workshop (e.g., readers theater) that allows students to use various character voices Making PVC phones available for students to use during reading times Leading a class lesson on changing voice during oral reading Strengthening diaphragm muscles using a whistle Providing a fake microphone for students to use during presentations as a visual reminder to speak loud enough for your audience
Fluency	Leading a guided reading group that allows students to reread texts to focus on fluency Practicing whole-class breathing techniques and strategies prior to oral communication Using digital books and having the student follow along in the print copy Reading a short section of a book aloud, then having the student immediately read it back to you, matching his or her voice to yours
Language	Making question prompts available during morning meeting Planning structured activities for students to have academic and personal conversations throughout the day Making picture cards available to students Making communication devices available for students Demonstrating and training other students in the class how to communicate with someone who uses augmentative and alternative communication Demonstrating breathing and meditation techniques for students to use before presentations Creating role plays that allow students to learn the social aspects of communication Providing professional development to all staff working with anyone who uses augmentative communication
Augmentative communication	Working in collaboration with your assistive technology specialist to select use of augmentative communication device Learning how to utilize each device, program individualized words and statements to support social interaction, and supporting educators to use within the context of general education
Record keeping	Documenting services to ensure accountability of therapy provision Keeping anecdotal records based on observations Generating data for use in response to intervention Reviewing individualized education program goals
Assessment	Administering, scoring, interpreting, and making recommendations based on assessment date Conducting clinical observations

Therapy Rooms

A *therapy room* is a place in which students are generally supposed to spend a short amount of time working on a specific skill, performance, or routine before returning to the LRE (e.g., general education classroom, lunch room, hallway).

Resource Rooms

A *resource room* is a place in which students are generally supposed to spend a short amount of time working on a specific skill or subject before returning to the general education classroom. The instruction in these classrooms is typically delivered in a small group with one educator teaching a small group of students or with one teacher working directly with one student.

Self-Contained Classrooms

A *self-contained classroom* is designed for instructing only students who have disabilities. The original purpose of this kind of classroom was to group students who had similar learning needs. These kinds of classrooms have become very controversial because students in self-contained classrooms interact on a very limited basis, if at all, with students who do not have disabilities.

Community-Based Instruction

Some SLPs work in community-based settings. The idea behind community-based instruction is that some students require instruction to prepare them for life in the community by working on job skills and independent living skills. Therefore, some students receive their instruction in the community. Some types of community-based locations include job sites, recreational facilities, grocery stores, or other community locations.

WHAT DOES A SPEECH-LANGUAGE PATHOLOGIST DO?

SLPs provide direct and indirect service delivery methods to meet the unique needs of students. Indirect service involves a collaborative or consultation approach whereby the SLP works with educators, other related service providers, parents, and other school staff to plan and implement intervention strategies across the educational environment. The SLP might also provide modeling or training to the adults. With this approach, other professionals may implement the intervention strategies that an SLP recommends. ASHA endorses the use of an integrated services model to deliver related services that is authentically embedded in specially designed instruction within the context of a student's school routine. The rationale is that skills can be learned and applied in natural situations within the LRE. Dunn (1990) found that similar levels of goal attainment can be made through consultation services and that this is a viable service provision method. Furthermore, this indirect consultation SLP role is supported by IDEA 2004, which stated that related services can be delivered to "the child, or on behalf of the child, and [as] program modifications and supports for school personnel" (U.S.C. 614[d][1][A][i][IV]). You may provide suggestions to teachers and parents to implement the use of communication devices, articulation practice, and pragmatic language development social groups, and may model techniques to staff. More suggestions for consultation recommendations are given throughout this book.

Direct service involves the SLP working with the student through facilitating a small group, through whole class instruction, or one-to-one. Direct service can be provided both through push-in and pull-out therapy. *Push-in,* or *integrated, services* means that an SLP provides intervention strategies within the child's natural learning environment. This intervention can be individual or group-based within the general education curriculum and context. *Pull-out services* are used to remediate a specific skill, pattern, or routine in an alternative room or school setting and can be conducted in a one-on-one or group format. In adherence to IDEA 2004 and best practices, we advocate for services to be conducted within the LRE, meaning the space where the activity, routine, skill, or need naturally occurs within the school environment, alongside grade-level peers.

COMMONLY ASKED QUESTIONS ABOUT THE ROLE OF SPEECH-LANGUAGE PATHOLOGISTS

Q. Does the professional organization ASHA support inclusive speech and language therapy provision?

A. The short answer is yes. ASHA recognizes that with the passage of IDEA 2004, the work of school-based SLPs has evolved. IDEA mandates that students with disabilities participate in, have access to, and progress in the general education curriculum or natural environment. See the discussion that highlights the transformation of an SLP's role from caseload to workload.

Q. What is wrong with pull-out speech and language therapy?

A. The purpose of school-based speech and language therapy is "to optimize individuals' ability to communicate and swallow, thereby improving quality of life" (ASHA, 2007). In other words, SLPs provide supports that help students communicate during their school day. Any skills, routines, activities, or performance tasks that students need to work on should be learned and practiced in their naturally occurring context. This is the LRE. Furthermore, students with disabilities have the right to learn and socialize alongside their grade-level peers. Pull-out provision of any kind of service or support has deleterious effects on one's self-esteem and ability to learn and disrupts a sense of belonging. Many therapists across the country are transforming their practices, and their therapy supports are now portable, meaning they can be delivered right in these naturally occurring contexts.

Q. Can I lead a small-group station in an inclusive classroom?

A. Yes, you can lead a small-group station within an inclusive classroom. Your station would be focused so that it provides a therapeutic intervention that is connected to the academic content of the classroom.

Q. Can I teach an entire class by myself?

A. An SLP can lead a whole-class lesson and have a purposeful co-teaching role. The general educator and therapist can work together to develop a co-teaching relationship and work as a team to deliver the therapeutic intervention and academic learning experiences. This works because there is a certified teacher in the room and the lesson was co-planned. See Chapter 4 for more information.

Q. Who is ultimately responsible for meeting the IEP goals of the student I work with?

A. The special education teacher, general education teacher, and related service providers assigned to the student are responsible. That is, the team of educators and therapists are jointly vested in ensuring that students with disabilities meet their independent education goals.

CONCLUSION

The SLP's role is vital to the lives and daily functioning of so many of our students. Understanding your roles and responsibilities is essential for you to do your job effectively. This chapter has provided a brief look at the history of inclusive education and the evolution of SLPs within education, discussed the roles and responsibilities of SLPs today, and provided answers to some commonly asked questions. As you can see, SLPs are related service providers who support students to benefit from special education services. The next chapter is designed to give you some background on special education.

NOTES

_____
_____
_____
_____
_____
_____
_____
_____
_____
_____
_____
_____
_____
_____
_____
_____
_____
_____
_____
_____
_____
_____
_____
_____
_____
_____

2

Special Education

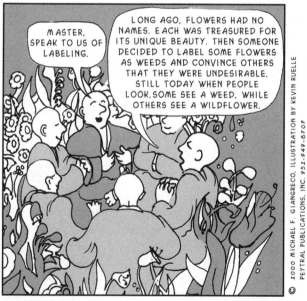

WHAT DO YOU CHOOSE TO SEE?
WEEDS OR WILDFLOWERS?

"I prefer to think of my disability as a type of diversity rather than deviance or deficiency: my disability is just one characteristic or attribute among many that make me who I am. People do not need to prove their worthiness. Obviously, what we are talking about here is a human rights issue. We need to establish the unconditional and inherent worthiness of people regardless of what combinations of diverse characteristics they present."

—Norman Kunc (Giangreco, 1996/2004, p. 35)

"When I went to school, I studied to be a speech-language pathologist. I expected to spend a lot of time working on issues of fluency, voice, or speech sound production . . . but never expected that so much time would be spent supporting students with severe and multiple disabilities. So many students on my caseload have complex communication disorders that require intensive support. So, feeding, swallowing, cognition, language production, and assistive technologies had to quickly become part of my daily practice. Understanding the wide variety of potential disabilities would have been so useful."

—Ann (SLP)

We begin with the question that many have asked when they began work in the speech-language pathology field. What is special education? In this chapter, we answer that question along with the following ones: Who receives special education? What does *disability* mean? Why should people be cautious of labels? What does special education terminology mean? What are the different categories of disabilities? At the end of this chapter, we also answer other commonly asked questions.

This chapter identifies the important concepts and ideas that are essential to understand for anyone in the field of special education or related service provision. By knowing this information, SLPs can understand the larger educational system of which they are part. However, we fully recognize that many seasoned SLPs have expertise on this topic, so feel free to move on to Chapter 3.

WHAT IS SPECIAL EDUCATION?

Simply put, *special education* is individualized instruction designed to meet the unique needs of certain students. This type of customized instruction may require a student to have accommodations or modifications to his or her class work. *Accommodations* are adaptations to the curriculum that do not fundamentally alter or lower standards (e.g., test location, student response method). *Modifications* are changes to the curriculum that do alter the expectations (e.g., changes to the course content, timing, or test presentation). Any student who receives special education services may receive specialized materials (e.g., digital books), services (e.g., speech and language services), equipment (e.g., a communication system), or different teaching strategies (e.g., visual notes) (IDEA, 2004, PL 108-446). For example, a student who is deaf may require the services of a sign language interpreter in order to participate in the classroom. A student who has autism may require specialized materials such as a visual schedule to prepare for the changing routines in the school day. A student with a learning disability may require additional reading instruction or extended time for completing written assignments.

Special education is a part of general education. It is a system of supports to help students learn the general education curriculum. The legal definition of special education under IDEA 2004 is "specially designed instruction, at no cost to the child's parents, to meet the needs of a student with a disability" (20 U.S.C. § 1401 [25]).

This definition recognizes that some children have difficulty learning, behaving, or physically engaging in general education and, because of such disabilities, need individualized supports to help them to build their skills and abilities to reach their full potential in school. These additional services are at no cost to families and are funded by the local, state, and federal governments.

WHAT ARE RELATED SERVICES?

One type of related service that can be offered to students is speech-language pathology. IDEA 2004 defines the term *related services* as follows:

> Transportation, and such developmental, corrective, and other supportive services (including speech-language pathology and audiology services, interpreting services, psychological services, physical and occupational therapy, recreation, including therapeutic recreation, social work services, school nurse services) designed to enable a child with a disability to receive a free appropriate public education as described in the individualized education program of the child, counseling services, including rehabilitation counseling, orientation and mobility services, and medical services . . . as may be required to assist a child with a disability to benefit from special education, and includes the early identification and assessment of disabling conditions in children. (20 U.S.C. § 1401 [602][26][A])

In other words, speech-language pathology is a related service that is available to allow students to benefit from special education.

SPECIAL EDUCATION AND SPEECH-LANGUAGE THERAPY ARE SERVICES, NOT PLACES

In the past, when the terms *special education* or *speech-language pathology* were used, a special place came to mind. People thought of a room, a school, or another separate place to which children with disabilities went to receive different therapy services and special education. This notion, however, is rapidly changing. Special education and related services are no longer limited to a specific location. It has been established that all children—including children with autism, severe disabilities, multiple disabilities, and emotional or behavioral disabilities—learn best in classroom settings with their general education peers (Causton-Theoharis & Theoharis, 2008; Peterson & Hittie, 2002). Special education and related services are portable services (e.g., help with reading, math, fine motor skills) that can be brought directly to individual children within general education contexts.

Special education occurs in general education classrooms all over the United States and the rest of the world. When students with disabilities are educated primarily in general education settings, this is called *inclusive education*. In inclusive classrooms, teachers, related service providers, and paraprofessionals should ensure that children with special needs are part of the general education curriculum, instruction, and social scene as much as possible within the LRE. The next chapter on inclusive education will describe more fully the concept of LRE.

WHO RECEIVES SPECIAL EDUCATION?

Every year, under IDEA 2004, more than 6.5 million students in the United States between the ages of 3 and 21 receive special education services (U.S. Department of Education, 2011). In other words, roughly 11% of all school-age children qualify for special education services because they have disabilities.

Under IDEA 2004, the definition of a student with a disability is "one who has certain disabilities and who, because of the impairment, needs special education and related services" (20 U.S.C. § 1401 [3]). Each student qualifies for special education because he or she has at least one type of disability. Each of the different types of disability is defined and described later in this chapter.

When one examines the population of students who receive special education, several disturbing trends appear in the areas of gender, socioeconomic status, and race. First, even though the numbers of males and females in the general school population are equal, the population receiving special education is roughly two-thirds male (U.S. Department of Education, 2007). Second, the poverty rate is proportionately much higher among students who qualify for special education than in the entire school population (U.S. Department of Education, 2007). Last, a disproportionate number of certain racial or ethnic groups are served in special education. For example, because African Americans make up 14% of the general population, one might assume that only 14% of students who qualify for special education would be African American (Turnbull, Turnbull, Shank, & Smith, 2004). In fact, African American students represent 44.9% of the total number of students labeled as having learning disabilities (U.S. Department of Education, 2007). Further, African American students are three times more likely than Caucasian students to receive special education and related services. SLPs should be cognizant of these national trends that reveal the demographics of students in special education.

WHAT DOES *DISABILITY* MEAN?

Disability categories are used to "classify and think about the problems developing children may encounter" (Contract Consultants, IAC, 1997, p. 8, as cited in Kluth, 2003). Understanding a student's label is only the beginning point in learning about a child. As the quote by Kunc at the beginning of this chapter poignantly reminds us, disability is one type of diversity, "one characteristic or attribute among many that make me who I am" (Giangreco, 1996/2004, p. 35). A disability label reveals nothing about the student's individual gifts, talents, and strengths. A disability is one of many parts of a student. A disability does not describe who a person is; it describes only one aspect of the person.

To illustrate this point, take a moment to write down five descriptors about yourself. What did you include? Julie might include descriptors about who she is in relation to others, or her profession, or personality traits. The list might include mother, professor, lover of nature, daughter, and outgoing. Chelsea would include the following: compassionate, spunky, educator, driven, and athlete. Note that our lists did not include any deficiencies. We do not think of ourselves generally as individuals who do not balance our checkbooks very well, for example. The same is true for any individual with a disability. That person's area of disability is one (possibly very small) part of who he or she is. As one therapist described to us, "the basic philosophy of this [school] is one of human potential and inclusion regardless of what any diagnosis, label, or testing looks like." Think of each student's human potential, strengths, and talents.

FROM A MEDICAL MODEL TO THE SOCIAL CONSTRUCTION OF DISABILITY

Traditionally, SLPs, special educators, and other school personnel have used a medical model construction of disability in which disability is seen as a fixed deficit that resides in the person. This has allowed for disability diagnosis and referral out of the general education classroom. The educational interventions are geared toward brining the student toward normalcy. The medical model creates a binary division between students with and students without disabilities, and professionals use the deficits as a rationale for providing separate educational placements. Throughout this book, it is clear that we explicitly challenge this construction of disability. We also recognize that you, too, have begun to rethink this medicalized view of disability and see an alternative social construction of disability that is created by social, cultural, and political aspects of our educational community.

It is important to recognize that people create disability categories and that those categories shift and change over time. Medical professionals, teachers, and researchers— along with the federal government—have created these categories, and they are not static; they do and have changed. An extreme example of how disability is constructed is that, at one point in time, to qualify as having an intellectual disability (ID; or *mental retardation,* as it was initially called in federal legislation), a person needed to have an IQ of 80 or below. In 1973, the federal government lowered the cutoff IQ score to 70 points or below. So, in essence, with the single stroke of a pen, hundreds of thousands of people were "cured" (Ashby, 2008; Blatt, 1987).

Once created, these categories are reinforced. In other words, people see mainly what they are looking for. Once a student is assigned a label, educators begin seeing the child through a different lens—the lens of disability. We have seen this process at work numerous times. For example, during a research project conducted in a third-grade classroom, all of the students were busy working and talking as they finished their art projects. The room was bustling and busy. Suddenly, the art teacher shouted, "Jamie, that is the last time!" The teacher walked to the chalkboard and wrote Jamie's name down. Nearly all of the students were talking, yet Jamie, who happens to have a label of emotional disturbance, was noticed for being too talkative or out of line. In reality, Jamie's behavior looked no different from that of many of the other students.

Disability categories are created, and then people determine who qualifies and who does not. Have you ever worked with someone who had a label but you really did not think he or she had a disability? Have you ever seen a student who did not qualify for special education even though you thought he or she might? Disability labels are not hard and fast rules that describe people; they are indicators of patterns of difficulty for individuals and are determined by the perceptions of other people.

LABELS: PROCEED WITH CAUTION

A disability label may have both positive and negative effects on an individual. On one hand, many believe labels to be helpful for defining a common language for parents and professionals. This common language allows students access to certain supports and services that they need. In a way, a label is the necessary first step toward certain services (including the services of an SLP).

On the other hand, there are real problems with the labeling or categorizing of individuals. Kliewer and Biklen stated that labeling students can be a "demeaning process frequently contributing to stigmatization and leading to social and educational isolation" (1996, p. 83). The use of and overreliance on disability labels poses many problems. Disability labels can lead to stereotyping by causing teachers to see certain students in one, and only one, way. Labeling tends to highlight the differences among people. For example, when a student is assigned a label, teachers, therapists, and paraprofessionals begin to notice the differences between that student and his or her peers. Labels can lead to poor self-esteem as students begin to see themselves differently because of such labels. Also, labels convey the impression of permanence, even though, in some cases, students are only "disabled" when they are in school. Unfortunately, labels give professionals a real sense of security. They allow professionals to believe that "disability categories are static, meaningful, and well understood when in fact they are none of these things" (Kluth, 2010, p. 7).

Throughout this book, we use the language that is most common to the current educational system. We are well aware, however, of the real problems and, at times, dangers of thinking about difference in these ways. Some people use the term *dis/ability* (with a slash) to indicate that all students should focus on their individual abilities. Although we prefer the word *dis/ability,* we are purposefully using the language most common to education and therapy so that readers can easily connect this information to other information from the field.

THE ALPHABET SOUP OF EDUCATIONAL TERMINOLOGY

Alphabet soup: that is how the use of acronyms in the field of special education sometimes sounds. Understanding the language of special education can take a long time. The following is an alphabetical listing of a range of educational terms that are often used as acronyms:

- AAC: augmentative and alternative communication
- ADD/ADHD: attention deficit disorder and/or attention-deficit/hyperactivity disorder
- ASD: autism spectrum disorder
- ASHA: American Speech-Language-Hearing Association
- AT: assistive technology
- BIP: behavior intervention plan
- CBI: community-based instruction
- CCC: Certificate of Clinical Competence
- COTA: certified occupational therapy assistant
- CST: child study team
- DS: Down syndrome
- EBD: emotional behavioral disturbance
- ED: emotional disturbance
- ESY: extended school year
- FAPE: free appropriate public education
- FBA: functional behavioral assessment
- HI: hearing impaired
- ID: intellectual disability
- IDEA: Individuals with Disabilities Education Improvement Act
- IEP: individualized education program
- LD: learning disability
- LRE: least restrictive environment
- NCLB: No Child Left Behind Act
- OHI: other health impairment
- OI: orthopedic impairment
- OT: occupational therapist
- PBS: positive behavior support
- PT: physical therapist
- RTI: response to intervention
- SLD: specific learning disability

- SLP: speech-language pathologist
- TBI: traumatic brain injury
- VI: visual impairment

FEDERALLY RECOGNIZED CATEGORIES OF DISABILITY

How many different categories of disability are you aware of? There are 13 federal categories of disability. Every student who receives special education services has received a formal label representing one of the 13 categories. Now, without looking ahead to the next paragraph, take a moment to jot down on a piece of paper as many of the disability categories as you can. Compare your list with the information provided in the next paragraph.

The categories of disability include the following: 1) autism, 2) deafblindness, 3) deafness, 4) emotional disturbance (ED), 5) hearing impairment, 6) intellectual disability (ID; formerly called *mental retardation*), 7) multiple disabilities, 8) orthopedic impairment (OI), 9) other health impairments (OHIs), 10) specific learning disabilities (SLDs), 11) speech and language impairments, 12) traumatic brain injury (TBI), and 13) visual impairment (VI), including blindness. In the following subsections, we include the IDEA 2004 definition for each; however, the most useful way to understand each disability is to listen carefully to the people who have been labeled with the disability and understand the disability deeply. Therefore, after each of the definitions, we include voices of people who have been labeled with each of the particular disabilities. These voices are not meant to be examples; one person cannot possibly represent the entire population of students who have the same disability. Note the differences between the legal definitions and the definitions that the people themselves use. It is interesting that the legal definitions focus on what students cannot do or the difficulties they have, whereas the student voices focus more on the gifts and abilities of each individual.

Autism

Autism is defined by law as a developmental disability that significantly affects verbal and nonverbal communication and social interaction and adversely affects educational performance; autism is generally evident before age 3. Characteristics often associated with autism are engaging in repetitive activities and stereotyped movements, resistance to change in daily routines or the environment, and unusual responses to sensory experiences (IDEA, 2004, 34 C.F.R. § 300.8 [c][1][i]).

A person who has autism and lives with it every day offered a quite different definition of the disability:

> Some aspects of autism may be good or bad depending only on how they are perceived. For example, hyperfocusing is a problem if you're hyperfocusing on your feet and miss the traffic light change. On the other hand, hyperfocusing is a great skill for working on intensive projects. This trait is particularly well suited to freelancers and computer work. I would never argue that autism is all good or merely a difference. I do find that my autism is disabling. However, that doesn't mean that it is all bad or that I mean I want to be someone else. (Molton, 2000)

Another individual with autism described it this way: "I believe Autism is a marvelous occurrence of nature, not a tragic example of the human mind gone wrong. In many cases, Autism can also be a kind of genius undiscovered" (O'Neill, 1999, p. 14, as cited in Kluth, 2010, p. 3).

Deafblindness

Deafblindness is defined by law as "concomitant [simultaneous] hearing and visual impairments, the combination of which causes such severe communication and other developmental and educational needs that they cannot be accommodated in special education programs solely for children with deafness or children with blindness" (IDEA, 2004, 34 C.F.R. § 300.8 [c][2]).

In other words, students with deafblindness have both hearing and visual impairments. The population of students with deafblindness constitutes only 0.0001% of the special education population. Therefore, most SLPs probably will not support someone with this disability label. Many people who are deaf and blind learn to use tactile sign, a form of sign language that is felt with the hands.

Helen Keller is one of the most famous examples of a person with deafblindness. She wrote very articulately about what it was like to live with this label in her autobiography entitled *The Story of My Life* (1903). One quote from Keller describes how she interacted with the world: "The best and most beautiful things in the world cannot be seen or even touched. They must be felt within the heart" (p. 6).

Deafness

Deafness is legally defined as "a hearing impairment so severe that a child's educational performance is adversely affected; people with deafness have difficulty, with or without amplification, in processing linguistic information" (IDEA, 2004, 34 C.F.R. § 300.8 [c][3]). Students who qualify for special education under the category of deafness typically use sign language. These individuals can gain access to the general education curriculum through the use of a sign language interpreter, through oral methods of speech reading, or by reading other people's lips and facial expressions. A deaf college student identified as Mavis shared her experiences of living as a deaf person:

> It is true. Every weekend, I ride my high quality road racing bicycle at high speeds (sometimes as fast as 40 mph on the flats) with a bunch of men from my bicycle club. I am the only deaf person in that 500 member club. I also enjoy going to the shooting range to fire handguns and socialize. (Mavis, 2003)

Emotional Disturbance

ED is legally defined as

> A condition exhibiting one or more of the following characteristics for a long period of time and to a marked degree that adversely affects a child's educational performance:
>
> a. An inability to learn that cannot be explained by intellectual, sensory, or health factors.
>
> b. An inability to build or maintain satisfactory interpersonal relationships with peers and teachers.

c. Inappropriate types of behavior or feelings under normal circumstances.

d. A general pervasive mood of unhappiness or depression.

e. A tendency to develop physical symptoms or fears associated with personal or school problems. (IDEA, 2004, 34 C.F.R. § 300.8 [c][4])

These students make up about 8% of the special education population (U.S. Department of Education, 2011). This category of disability relates to how students behave. For a student to qualify for this category of disability, the student's behavior should look significantly different from that of peers (Taylor, Smiley, & Richards, 2009). Kerri, who has ED, described it this way:

> I misinterpret half of what [people] say to me and translate it to mean they don't want to be my friend anymore. Why should they? I am not worth their time or love or attention. Then I get angry with them and I turn on them. Hurt them before they can hurt me. It is so stupid, and I realize it later, but only after it is too late. ("Information on Bipolar," n.d.)

Hearing Impairment

Being identified as having a *hearing impairment* means that there is "an impairment in hearing, whether permanent or fluctuating, that adversely affects a child's educational performance but that is not included under the definition of deafness" (IDEA, 2004, 34 C.F.R. § 300.8 [c][5]). Students who have hearing impairments generally do not use sign language, because the hearing that they do have is useful to them. Instead, they might use an amplification system. One individual (Sarahjane Thompson) with a hearing impairment described her experience:

> The way I tend to explain [hearing impairment] is that it's not necessarily that you can't hear the words that people are using, it's that you hear sounds that resemble words, but you can't quite figure out what the sounds are. Like when a hearing person only just hears something, and asks someone to repeat themselves. Like that. Except for me it's way more frequent. So that's why I tend to use other strategies to figure out what's going on. I lip-read. . . . But lip-reading isn't perfect. A lot of the words look the same and so it's hard for me to use it exclusively to talk to someone. I tend to guess a lot. I'll catch most of a sentence and then sort of try to fill in the gaps myself. Usually it works. Sometimes it doesn't. . . . Every now and then I'll mis-hear an entire sentence and my brain will fill in the random words that sort of fit the syllables and sounds, but together those words do not make sense at all. . . . It's just so normal for me to be hearing impaired. People ask me what it's like to be [hearing impaired] and I just don't have a perfect answer for them. "What's it like to be able to hear?" There's no real comparison and so I don't really know what is different about it. Obviously hearing people can hear more and understand more sounds, but what does that mean? It can be really hard to explain. It's all about perception. (Williams & Thompson, 2008)

Intellectual Disability

The ID label is legally assigned to students who have "significantly subaverage general intellectual functioning, existing concurrently with impairments in adaptive behavior and manifested during the developmental period, that adversely affects a child's educational performance" (IDEA, 2004, 34 C.F.R. § 300.8 [c][6]). The term *mental retardation* is cited in IDEA 2004, but was changed in 2010 under Rosa's Law (PL 111-256,

2010) to *intellectual disability*. The definition, however, did not change. Another term commonly used is *cognitive disability*. This category constitutes 8.86% of students receiving special education services (U.S. Department of Education, 2011). People with ID vary greatly. Some students have speech and can write, whereas other students do not use speech and are unable to write. Lacking the ability to write or speak, however, does not mean that the person has no ideas or no desire to communicate with others. These students tend to deeply desire connections with others and, when given the tools to communicate, engage with other students and with the content.

The following is a first-person account from someone labeled with cognitive disabilities:

> What I would like is for you to understand that my biggest problem is not a neurological dysfunction. It is being misunderstood by people who think my problems are due to poor parenting. My mom has really tried to teach me proper social behaviors, but it just does not click all the time. Sometimes I can't remember the social rules. (FAS Community Resource Center, 2008)

This extract from Schalock and Braddock (2002) places among broader context Ollie Webb's words about her life with ID:

> I was often the target of cruel jokes. It was easy to take advantage of me. People called me retarded . . . I worked out there—17 years—and I made salads, sandwiches, and soup, and washed pots and pans. You name it, I done it out there. . . . One time I came in and the boss said, "I am going to take you off of salads." I said, "Why?" He said, "Cause you can't read." I said, "It make no difference. I can make salads and sandwiches." I said, "It make no damn difference." . . . It came time to leave the sad word retarded [to history]. . . . To say that people should be known by their names [and accomplishments], not by their disabilities, I ain't different from you. I am the same as you. I got a name, and I want you to call me by my name. My name is Ollie . . . Webb. (pp. 55–57)

Multiple Disabilities

The term *multiple disabilities* is legally defined as concomitant impairments (e.g., ID–blindness, ID–OI), the combination of which causes such severe educational needs that the student cannot be accommodated in a special educational setting solely for one of the impairments. The term does not include deafblindness (IDEA, 2004, 34 C.F.R. § 300.8 [c][7]). Roughly 2% of the special education population is considered to have multiple disabilities (U.S. Department of Education, 2011). Therefore, it is unlikely that you will work with someone who has that label.

Orthopedic Impairments

The term *orthopedic impairment* means a severe OI that adversely affects a child's educational performance. The term includes impairments caused by congenital impairments (e.g., clubfoot, absence of a body part), impairments caused by disease (e.g., poliomyelitis, bone tuberculosis), and impairments from other causes (e.g., cerebral palsy, amputations, fractures or burns that cause contractures) (IDEA, 2004, 34 C.F.R. § 300.8 [c][8]).

Angela Gabel, a high school student with cerebral palsy who uses a wheelchair, described herself and her experience in school as follows:

When you see me, I think the first thing you would notice is that I'm a pretty positive person. I love to listen to music, go horseback riding, and draw. . . . When I was in elementary school . . . I had friends and liked to play the same games as everyone else, but the teachers were always worried that I was too fragile and would hurt myself. (Gabel, 2006, p. 35)

Other Health Impairment

Other health impairment is legally defined as having limited strength, vitality, or alertness to environmental stimuli, resulting in limited alertness with respect to the educational environment, that

(a) is due to chronic or acute health problems such as asthma, attention deficit disorder or attention deficit hyperactivity disorder, diabetes, epilepsy, a heart condition, hemophilia, lead poisoning, leukemia, nephritis, rheumatic fever, and sickle cell anemia; and (b) adversely affects a child's educational performance. (IDEA, 2004, 34 C.F.R. § 300.8 [c][9])

This impairment includes students who have ADHD. The label *ADHD* is assigned to students who have difficulty maintaining attention, knowing when to slow down, or organizing themselves to finish tasks (American Psychiatric Association, 2000). Obviously, not everyone who has each of these disorders qualifies for special education, but if such a condition has been diagnosed by a medical professional and adversely affects a student's educational performance (and if the student needs additional supports), he or she is likely to qualify.

Jonathan Mooney, an author and public speaker with ADHD and dyslexia, explained his disability:

I have the attention span of a gnat. When I am forced to sit in a desk. . . . My mind wanders a little bit. I start to bounce my foot. I get called inattentive. What happens the moment I can get up? The moment I can move around? . . . How disabled am I at that moment of time? Not at all. (Mooney, 2007)

This impairment includes students who may have a repaired cleft palate, language disorders, voice disorders, swallowing disorders, and respiratory problems that impact speech production. The SLP might work with several students who fall under this larger category.

Specific Learning Disabilities

An SLD is legally defined as a disorder in one or more of the basic psychological processes involved in understanding or using spoken or written language; it may manifest itself in an imperfect ability to listen, think, speak, read, write, spell, or do mathematical calculations. The term includes such conditions as perceptual disabilities, brain injury, minimal brain dysfunction, dyslexia, and developmental aphasia. The term does not include learning problems that are primarily the results of visual, hearing, or motor disabilities; of ID; of ED; or of environmental, cultural, or economic disadvantages (IDEA, 2004, 34 C.F.R. § 300.8 [c][10]).

Almost half of all students categorized as having disabilities fall under this category. This is the most frequently occurring disability; thus, you are quite likely to work with students who have the label of SLD.

In an article about being a student with a learning disability, Caitlin Norah Callahan wrote her advice to others:

I believe one key idea is to find one's own definition of the dual identity within oneself as a learner and as a student. The learner is the one who makes an effort to be curious, involved and motivated. Not all knowledge is taught in school. It is the student identity that gets labeled as the disabled. The "learning disability" should not be allowed to overwhelm one's desire to attain knowledge. The learner in you must prevent it. (Callahan, 1997)

Speech and Language Impairment

Speech and language impairment is legally defined as a communication disorder such as stuttering, impaired articulation, a language impairment, or a voice impairment that adversely affects a child's educational performance (IDEA, 2004, 34 C.F.R. § 300.8 [c][11]).

This is the second most common disability category. Approximately 19% of students who qualify for special education are served under this category (U.S. Department of Education, 2011). Students who qualify for this disability have a wide range of impairment. Some students who receive speech and language services have difficulty with articulation or fluency (e.g., stuttering). Other students might not use speech.

The following is a story from a person who did not have speech in his early years but who later was able to communicate through the use of a communication system. This story illustrates the frustration inherent in not having a reliable method of speech:

> I know what it is like to be fed potatoes all my life. After all potatoes are a good basic food for everyday, easy to fix in many different ways. I hate potatoes! But then who knew that but me? I know what it is like to be dressed in reds and blues when my favorite colors are mint greens, lemon yellows, and pinks. I mean really can you imagine [what it is like not to communicate]? Mama found me one night curled up in a ball in my bed crying, doubled over in pain. I couldn't explain to her where or how I hurt. So, after checking me over the best she could, she thought I had a bad stomachache due to constipation. Naturally, a quick cure for that was an enema. It did not help my earache at all! (Paul-Brown & Diggs, 1993, p. 8)

Traumatic Brain Injury

TBI is legally defined as an acquired injury to the brain caused by an external physical force, resulting in total or partial functional disability or psychosocial impairment, or both, that adversely affects a child's educational performance. The term applies to open or closed head injuries resulting in impairments in one or more areas, such as cognition; language; memory; attention; reasoning; abstract thinking; judgment; problem solving; sensory, perceptual, and motor abilities; psychosocial behavior; physical functions; information processing; and speech. The term does not include brain injuries that are congenital, degenerative, or induced by birth trauma (IDEA, 2004, 34 C.F.R. § 300.8 [c][12]).

This type of disability differs from the others because it is acquired during the person's lifetime (e.g., car accident or blow to the head). People are not born with this condition—instead, they acquire the disability. The emotional adjustment to acquiring a disability is an issue not only for the student but also for parents or guardians and teachers, therapists, and other members of the educational team.

A teenager who endured a traumatic brain injury reflected on what she saw as her new life:

> The three-month coma that followed and the years of rehabilitation are only a blur to me. I slowly awoke over the next two years becoming aware of my surroundings as well as myself and my

inabilities, one being that I could no longer sing as I was left with a severe speech impediment. (Parker, 2008)

Visual Impairment, Including Blindness

A VI is legally defined as an impairment in vision that, even with correction, adversely affects a child's educational performance. The term includes both partial sight and blindness (IDEA, 2004, 34 C.F.R. § 300.8 [c][13]).

The services received by students under this category of disability differ depending on the severity or type of VI. Some students with VIs use magnifiers and larger print texts; students who have no vision receive mobility training (or training on how to walk around their environment) and instruction in how to read braille.

Distribution of Students with Disabilities in Each Category

How many students qualify for each of the different types of disabilities? The pie graph shown in Figure 2.1 depicts the percentages of students receiving special education services from ages 6 to 21 and the percentages of students who fall under each of the categories of disabilities. As Figure 2.1 indicates, the high-incidence (or

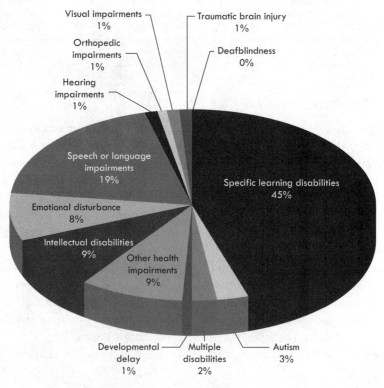

Figure 2.1. Percent distribution of students with disabilities. (*Source:* Data Accountability Center, n.d.)

most common) disabilities are learning disabilities, speech and language disabilities, ID, and other health impairment. The rest of the categories are considered low incidence (or not as common).

Now that you have read through each of the definitions of disabilities, we reiterate the importance of knowing these definitions, but keep in mind that this is only a (very small) step in understanding a student. Chapter 5 focuses more on how to think about students in general, with very little focus on individual disabilities.

COMMONLY ASKED QUESTIONS ABOUT SPECIAL EDUCATION

Q. How can I learn about the students I am supporting?

A. Start by reading each student's IEP and talking to the student and his or her parents. You can also get to know the student by asking questions about his or her likes, dislikes, interests, and struggles.

Here are some questions that would be helpful when getting to know a student:

- What do you want me to know about you?
- What do you like about school?
- What do you not like about school?
- What do you enjoy doing outside of school?
- Would you tell me about your friends?
- How do you prefer to be supported?
- What do you need from me?
- What do you not want me to do?

You can also ask the teacher about the strengths and needs of the student. Here are some good questions you could ask:

- What is motivating for this student?
- What does this student enjoy?
- Would you tell me about this student's friends?
- How can we support this student's social needs?
- What are this student's academic needs?
- How can we best support this student's academic needs?
- Does this student have challenging behavior?
- How can we best support this student's behavior?

- Does this student have sensory needs that I should be aware of?

- Does this student have communication needs that I might need to know?

- What modifications does this student use?

- Does this student use assistive technology?

- What else do I need to know about this student?

Q.   I have a student with a unique disability who receives speech-language pathology services. Where can I get more training about how to effectively work with this student?

A.   You should ask. Start with your building principal or the head of special education in your school. The following elements could be included in an e-mail, phone call, or letter to your supervisors:

- Be specific about the type of training you need. For example, you could say, "In my current position, I need to know more about working with students with autism who communicate using nonverbal gestures and augmentative communication systems."

- Ask whether they know of any training that is being offered, or find a conference to attend that features training about the disability, or ask whether the school could hire an educational consultant to work with the school or team.

CONCLUSION

Understanding disability is critical to understanding the larger systems of special education and related service provision. Nonetheless, the only way to truly understand certain individual students is to get to know people who live with those disabilities. In addition, developing an authentic relationship with the individual is the best way to understand that person's strengths, interests, talents, and needs. Reading the definitions of the 13 federal categories of disability is just the first step to understanding the students you support.

Having covered some of the basics of special education, we commence the joyful work of helping you to learn about individual students and helping to support them in the classroom. Chapter 3 focuses on including students with disabilities.

NOTES

_____
_____
_____
_____
_____
_____
_____
_____
_____
_____
_____
_____
_____
_____
_____
_____
_____
_____
_____
_____
_____
_____
_____
_____
_____

3

Inclusive Education

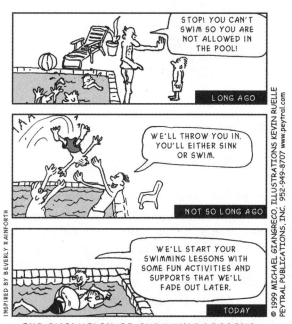

THE EVOLUTION OF SWIMMING LESSONS:
SURPRISINGLY SIMILAR TO THE EVOLUTION
OF INCLUDING STUDENTS WITH
DISABILITIES IN GENERAL EDUCATION.

"I was supporting Mike in his math class—he types to communicate. I realized that support is so much more complex in the general education classroom. I had to not only position my body to best support his typing, but also help him respond to the fast-paced questions that the teacher was asking. I also had to consider my own voice volume and prompts, so that I was being quiet and not distracting him from the teacher's directions, I had to consider the other students at the table who were also interacting with Mike and help him respond. This way he could really be part of the entire class. It is different than being in the speech and language room. I absolutely think it [inclusive support] is much better for him."

—Kathryn (SLP)

As you can see in Kathryn's vignette, she thinks that providing communication support within the general education classroom is better for the student. In this chapter, we identify the concepts necessary to understanding inclusive education, such as belonging, the history of inclusive education, major legal concepts, the definition of inclusive education, indicators of inclusive education, IEPs, and commonly asked questions.

BELONGING

"To be rooted is perhaps the most important and least recognized need of the human soul."

—Simone Weil (2001)

One central reason that students are being included in general education settings is that every child, with or without disabilities, has the right to belong. All human beings desire friendships, relationships, and academic challenge. Students with disabilities are no different.

Think for a moment about yourself. Think of a time you believed that you truly belonged somewhere. Was it a group, a club, a sports team, or a work environment? Now think about your behavior in that setting. How did you behave? How did you feel? If someone looked at you, how did you act? Most people are more willing to take risks, to contribute, to share, and to learn in such environments. When you feel connected to a group of people, you are likely more talkative, more engaged, and more willing to be yourself. The same is true for children.

Now, on the contrary, think of a time that you believed you did not belong or were ostracized from a group. How did you behave? How did you feel? In those situations, many people respond by being withdrawn and quiet, shutting themselves off from the group. Or, a person might respond by leaving the situation or getting angry. The same is true for children in school. It is essential to feel connected to a group or part of the school community. Not only is this important for self-worth, but it is also important for learning.

When working with a group of teachers, therapists, and paraprofessionals, we asked the preceding questions. Their responses are shown in Table 3.1.

Table 3.1. Feelings associated with inclusion and exclusion

When I was included	When I was excluded
I felt loved	I was angry
I felt cared for	I was withdrawn
I took risks	I was quiet
I felt smart	I was hurt
I was myself	I cried
I laughed often	I felt sick
I was creative	I did not participate
I was open to learn	I tried to leave the group

Examine the responses shown in the table. How do they relate to students in school? Have you seen students in school who feel sick, angry, withdrawn, or hurt? Have you seen students who behave in ways that let you know they do not believe that they belong? On the other hand, have you noticed students who are engaged, acting like themselves, and freely taking risks? As teachers, we have observed students who regularly felt connected and those who did not. Helping students feel that they belong is one of the most important jobs of the educational team.

If a system of special education excludes and places children in rooms, hallways, or schools that are separate from the general education population, they will not behave as well or learn as well. School administrators, therapists, and teachers all over the country are rethinking the practice of isolating students with disabilities in one room and pulling students out for services (Causton-Theoharis & Theoharis, 2008; McLeskey & Waldron, 2006). Isolating students in this way causes them to feel different from everyone else and not part of the larger school community. This type of segregation has real consequences for students' self-esteem and ability to learn (Peterson & Hittie, 2002). Inclusive education was built on the foundation that all people have the basic human right to belong.

THE HISTORY OF INCLUSIVE EDUCATION

You might have attended a school in which students with disabilities were educated down the hall, in a separate wing, or in a separate school. You also might have attended a school in which you sat beside kids with disabilities. Your own schooling experience shapes your personal thoughts about inclusive education.

Before 1975, students with disabilities did not have the legal right to attend school. As a result, many students with more significant disabilities were educated in separate schools (paid for by their parents) or institutions; some were not educated at all. In 1975, Congress passed the Education for All Handicapped Children Act (PL 94-142), which has since been reauthorized, most recently as IDEA 2004 (PL 108-446). This law, which guarantees all students with disabilities the right to a public education, has proved a major step forward for people with disabilities and their families. This law ensures that all students with disabilities have access to FAPE in the LRE. Each of these terms is defined in the next section. Because speech-language pathology is a service meant to allow students to benefit from special education, special education laws are very important to understand.

Free Appropriate Public Education

In order to explain what is meant by *free appropriate public education,* consider each term separately:

Free: All students with disabilities have the right to attend school and the supports and services necessary to their education will be paid for at the public expense.

Appropriate: All students with disabilities must be provided the assistive technology, aids, and services that allow them to participate in academic and nonacademic activities.

Public education: This education is guaranteed in a public school setting.

Least Restrictive Environment

The terminology that is used to support inclusion in the law is *LRE*. This term is explicitly cited in IDEA 2004, which stipulates that all students with disabilities have the legal right to be placed in the LRE.

LRE means that, to the maximum extent appropriate, a school district must educate any student with a disability in the regular classroom with appropriate aids and supports, referred to as *supplementary aids and services,* along with the student's peers without disabilities, in the school he or she would attend if the student did not have a disability (IDEA, 2004).

Under LRE, the general education classroom is the first place to be considered for placing a student with a disability before more restrictive options are considered. In other words, services should first be provided in the general education classroom.

What Are Supplementary Aids and Services?

In the law, SLPs are to help students not only benefit from special education, but also gain access to supplementary aids and services. Supplementary aids and services that educators have successfully used include modifications to the regular class curriculum (e.g., preferential seating, use of a computer, taped lectures, reduced seat time), assistance of a teacher with special education training, special education training for the regular teacher, use of computer-assisted devices, provision of notetakers, and changes to materials. See Figure 3.1 for a long checklist of supplementary aids and services. We include such a long list of supplementary aids and services because the important point here is that all of this must be tried before considering removal from the general education classroom.

Educators must utilize all of the possible supplementary aids and services before determining that a student can leave the general education classroom. Inclusion is

Checklist of Sample
Supplemental Supports, Aids, and Services

Directions: When considering the need for personalized supports, aids, or services for a student, use this checklist to help identify which supports will be the least intrusive, only as special as necessary, and the most natural to the context of the classroom.

Environmental	
	Preferential seating
	Planned seating ___ Bus ___ Classroom ___ Lunchroom ___ Auditorium ___ Other
	Alter physical room arrangement. (Specify: _____.)
	Use study carrels or quiet areas.
	Define area concretely (e.g., carpet squares, tape on floor, rug area).
	Reduce/minimize distractions. ___ Visual ___ Spatial ___ Auditory ___ Movement
	Teach positive rules for use of space.
Pacing of Instruction	
	Extend time requirements.
	Vary activity often.
	Allow breaks.
	Omit assignments requiring copying in timed situations.

Figure 3.1. Checklist of Sample Supplemental Supports, Aids, and Services.

(continued)

Republished with permission of Sage Publications, from Villa, R.A., Thousand, J.S., & Nevin, A.I. (2008). *A guide to co-teaching: Practical tips for facilitating learning* (2nd ed., pp. 169–171). Thousand Oaks, CA: Corwin Press; permission conveyed through Copyright Clearance Center, Inc.

In *The Speech-Language Pathologist's Handbook for Inclusive School Practices* by Julie Causton and Chelsea P. Tracy-Bronson (2014, Paul H. Brookes Publishing Co., Inc.)

Figure 3.1. *(continued)* (page 2 of 7)

	Send additional copy of the text home for summer preview.
	Provide home set of materials for preview or review.

Presentation of Subject Matter

	Teach to the student's learning style/strength intelligences. ___ Verbal/Linguistic ___ Logical/Mathematical ___ Visual/Spatial ___ Naturalist ___ Bodily/Kinesthetic ___ Musical ___ Interpersonal ___ Intrapersonal
	Use active, experiential learning.
	Use specialized curriculum.
	Record class lectures and discussions to replay later.
	Use American Sign Language and/or total communication.
	Provide prewritten notes, an outline, or an organizer (e.g., mind map).
	Provide a copy of classmate's notes (e.g., use NCR paper, photocopy).
	Use functional and meaningful application of academic skills.
	Present demonstrations and models.
	Use manipulatives and real objects in mathematics.
	Highlight critical information or main ideas.
	Preteach vocabulary.
	Make and use vocabulary files or provide vocabulary lists.
	Reduce the language level of the reading assignment.
	Use facilitated communication.

(continued)

Figure 3.1. *(continued)*   (page 3 of 7)

	Use visual organizers/sequences.
	Use paired reading/writing.
	Reduce seat time in class or activities.
	Use diaries or learning logs.
	Reword/rephrase instructions and questions.
	Preview and review major concepts in primary language.
Materials	
	Limit amount of material on page.
	Record texts and other class materials.
	Use study guides and advanced organizers.
	Use supplementary materials.
	Provide note-taking assistance.
	Copy class notes.
	Scan tests and class notes into computer.
	Use large print.
	Use braille material.
	Use communication book or board.
	Provide assistive technology and software (e.g., Intelli-Talk).
Specialized Equipment or Procedure	
	___ Wheelchair ___ Walker ___ Standing board ___ Positioning ___ Computer ___ Computer software ___ Electronic typewriter

(continued)

Figure 3.1. *(continued)*   *(page 4 of 7)*

	___ Video ___ Modified keyboard ___ Voice synthesizer ___ Switches ___ Augmentative communication device ___ Catheterization ___ Suctioning ___ Braces ___ Restroom equipment ___ Customized mealtime utensils, plates, cups, and other materials

Assignment Modification

	Give directions in small, distinct steps (written/picture/verbal).
	Use written backup for oral directions.
	Use pictures as supplement to oral directions. ___ Lower difficulty level. ___ Raise difficulty level. ___ Shorten assignments. ___ Reduce paper-and-pencil tasks.
	Read or record directions to the student(s).
	Give extra cues or prompts.
	Allow student to record or type assignments.
	Adapt worksheets and packets.
	Use compensatory procedures by providing alternate assignments when demands of class conflict with student capabilities.
	Ignore spelling errors/sloppy work.
	Ignore penmanship.

Self-Management/Follow-Through

	Provide pictorial or written daily or weekly schedule.
	Provide student calendars.

(continued)

Figure 3.1. (continued)   (page 5 of 7)

	Check often for understanding/review.
	Request parent reinforcement.
	Have student repeat directions.
	Teach study skills.
	Use binders to organize material.
	Design/write/use long-term assignment time lines.
	Review and practice real situations.
	Plan for generalization by teaching skill in several environments.

Testing Adaptations

	Provide oral instructions and/or read test questions.
	Use pictorial instructions/questions.
	Read test to student.
	Preview language of test questions.
	Ask questions that have applications in real settings.
	Administer test individually. ___ Use short answer. ___ Use multiple choice. ___ Shorten length. ___ Extend time frame. ___ Use open-note/open-book tests.
	Modify format to reduce visual complexity or confusion.

Social Interaction Support

	Use natural peer supports and multiple, rotating peers.
	Use peer advocacy.
	Use cooperative learning group.

(continued)

Republished with permission of Sage Publications, from Villa, R.A., Thousand, J.S., & Nevin, A.I. (2008). *A guide to co-teaching: Practical tips for facilitating learning* (2nd ed., pp. 169–171). Thousand Oaks, CA: Corwin Press; permission conveyed through Copyright Clearance Center, Inc.

In *The Speech-Language Pathologist's Handbook for Inclusive School Practices* by Julie Causton and Chelsea P. Tracy-Bronson (2014, Paul H. Brookes Publishing Co., Inc.)

Figure 3.1. *(continued)* (page 6 of 7)

	Institute peer tutoring.
	Structure opportunities for social interaction (e.g., Circle of Friends).
	Focus on social process rather than end product.
	Structure shared experiences in school and extracurricular activities.
	Teach friendship, sharing, and negotiation skills to classmates.
	Teach social communication skills. ___ Greetings ___ Conversation ___ Turn taking ___ Sharing ___ Negotiation ___ Other

Level of Staff Support (Consider *after* considering previous categories)

	Consultation
	Stop-in support
	Team teaching (parallel, supportive, complementary, or co-teaching)
	Daily in-class staff support
	Total staff support (staff are in close proximity)
	One-to-one assistance
	Specialized personnel support (if indicated, identify time needed)

Support		Time Needed
	Instructional support assistant	
	Health care assistant	
	Behavior assistant	

(continued)

In *The Speech-Language Pathologist's Handbook for Inclusive School Practices* by Julie Causton and Chelsea P. Tracy-Bronson
(2014, Paul H. Brookes Publishing Co., Inc.)

Figure 3.1.   *(continued)*   *(page 7 of 7)*

	Signing assistant	
	Nursing	
	Occupational therapy	
	Physical therapy	
	Speech-language pathologist	
	Augmentative communication specialist	
	Transportation	
	Counseling	
	Adaptive physical education	
	Transition planning	
	Orientation/mobility	
	Career counseling	

In *The Speech-Language Pathologist's Handbook for Inclusive School Practices* by Julie Causton and Chelsea P. Tracy-Bronson
(2014, Paul H. Brookes Publishing Co., Inc.)

not mentioned in the law, but it is implied, and people use LRE and the multitude of supplementary aids and services to support the idea of inclusion. Therefore, inclusion has been defined by scholars.

DEFINING INCLUSIVE EDUCATION

"I believe they thought they knew the best destination for me, but they were mistaken. The more naive therapist often perceived the destination as being one of normalcy: to make me more valuable in society's eyes. This may not even have been conscious to the therapists: I think it may have been unconscious."

—Norman Kunc (Giangreco, 1996/2004)

Kunc defined *inclusive education* as

The valuing of diversity within the human community. When inclusive education is fully embraced, we abandon the idea that children have to become "normal" in order to contribute to the world. . . . We begin to look beyond typical ways of becoming valued members of the community, and in doing so, begin to realize the achievable goal of providing all children with an authentic sense of belonging. (1992, p. 20)

Udvari-Solner used another definition of inclusion:

Inclusive schooling propels a critique of contemporary school culture and thus, encourages practitioners to reinvent what can be and should be to realize more humane, just and democratic learning communities. Inequities in treatment and educational opportunity are brought to the forefront, thereby fostering attention to human rights, respect for difference and value of diversity. (1997, p. 142)

WHAT DOES INCLUSION LOOK LIKE? INDICATORS OF INCLUSIVE CLASSROOMS

Some indicators of inclusive schooling environments include natural proportions, team teaching, community building, differentiation, access, and engaging instruction.

Natural Proportions

In any one classroom, the number of students with disabilities should reflect the natural population of students with disabilities in the school (i.e., no more than 12%). For example, if students with disabilities comprise 12% of the natural school population, then no more than 12% of its students in any one of its classrooms should have a disability. In an inclusive classroom, half the class will not be made up of students with disabilities. Having a greater number of students with disabilities clustered in one setting increases the density of need, making the class more like a special education setting.

Team Teaching

Inclusive classrooms often have two teachers (one general and one special education teacher) with equitable responsibilities for educating all the students. Related service providers often co-teach or teach small groups in the general education classroom. Or else, they provide consulting to the teachers or to the paraprofessional, so that a student's therapy goals can be met seamlessly in the general education classroom.

Community Building

In inclusive classrooms, educators continually use community building to ensure that students feel connected to one another and to their teachers. A common theme in community building is that different people learn in different ways. Community building approaches vary, but, in an inclusive classroom, the day may start out with a morning meeting at which students share their feelings or important life events. You might see organized community building in which students learn about each other in systematic ways. For example, the students might be doing a community-building exercise called "Homework in a Bag"; in this exercise, each student brings one item that represents him- or herself and shares the item with a small group of other students. Many therapists help to lead these community-building activities, as students' social needs are often met by SLPs.

Differentiation

In an inclusive classroom, it is clear that learners of various academic, social, and behavioral levels and needs share one learning environment. Therefore, the content, process, or product is differentiated. Students might work on similar goals, but they do so in different ways. For example, all students might be working on math problems, with some using manipulatives, some drawing out their answers, some checking their problems on calculators, and some using wipe-off markers and whiteboards. SLPs are often key players in planning for meaningful differentiation that meets both academic and communication skills.

Students Do Not Leave to Learn

An inclusive classroom does not have a virtual revolving door of students leaving for specialized instruction in a specific skill. Therapies and services occur within the context of the general education classroom. For example, instead of the student going to a small room with an SLP to work on voice volume and answering questions, the SLP works with the general education teacher to find an appropriate time where students will be working in partners and questioning each other. Together they design the questionnaire that all of the students will use. The SLP comes to the classroom at that point during the lesson and supports the student to answer questions loudly enough for the partner to hear. She also suggests that the student get a copy of the questionnaire the night before so he or she can plan out answers. One of the key features of inclusive schooling is that students are not removed from the classroom for remediation. Instead, services and supports are brought directly to them.

Engaging Instruction

Inclusive classrooms do not entail a lot of large-group lectures in which the teachers talk and the students passively sit and listen. Learning is engaging and exciting in inclusive classrooms. Teachers plan instruction with the range of learning styles in mind. In inclusive classrooms, students experience active learning; they often are up and out of their seats, with partner work and group work used frequently. The content is planned to meet the needs of students to move around, to work with others, to engage in communication, to physically touch and interact with the content. Learning experiences are designed to incorporate multiple sensory modalities. Inclusive classrooms are natural places to incorporate specific speech and language skills.

WHY SHOULD I PROVIDE SERVICES WITHIN INCLUSIVE CLASSROOMS?

The first reason for providing speech-language pathology services within the inclusive classrooms is that the law supports it (IDEA, 2004; NCLB, 2001). A second reason is that the major national organization for SLPs, ASHA, clearly supports inclusive services and collaborative service delivery. Third, students tend to perform much better academically when they are educated alongside their peers and not removed from the general education classroom. In part, this is because when they are pulled out, they miss significant portions of the classroom content. Last, it is likely that the students being pulled out are the least likely to be able to handle multiple transitions each day. Providing inclusive speech and language therapy not only allows therapists to follow the spirit of the law and the intention of ASHA, but also provides the best educational setting for students to maximize their academic and social potential.

HOW DOES INCLUSIVE EDUCATION FIT WITH RESPONSE TO INTERVENTION?

Schools and districts across the country have adopted the response to intervention (RTI) triangle model: the base of the triangle is good curriculum and instruction, then some students are given prescribed intervention, and fewer students receive additional and even more focused intervention. The benefits of RTI include universal assessment and screening of all students, quality instruction matched to specific educational needs, frequent monitoring, and a schoolwide approach to using data to make decisions for related services and educational interventions (Ehren, Montgomery, Rudebusch, &

Whitmire, 2013). Authentic inclusive education is a way to significantly expand the base of the triangle to allow many students who typically struggle in that base to be more successful. It is important to recognize that the schools that embrace inclusive education are seeing positive results for students who typically receive interventions in more restrictive settings.

For SLPs, RTI offers an opportunity to contribute unique expertise to monitoring, intervention, and assessment practices. As Ehren and colleagues explained, "SLPs offer expertise in the language basis of literacy and learning, experience with collaborative approaches to instruction/intervention, and an understanding of the use of student outcomes data when making instructional decisions" (Ehren et al., 2013, p. 1). With expertise in language, the related disorders and disabilities, and appropriate interventions, SLPs offer vital contributions in serving as intervention team members, creating and conducting progress-monitoring systems that are used throughout the school, consulting with educators about initial interventions in the RTI tiers, and assisting families to understand their child's language challenges and progress (Ehren et al., 2013). SLPs continue to play critical roles in using multiple assessments to identify students with speech-language disabilities, determining appropriate services and making recommendations to the RTI team, and collaborating with educators to provide services for students with communication disabilities (Ehren et al., 2013).

Whereas some schools are looking for the prescriptive intervention to be delivered to a targeted group of students, inclusive education can offer a way to provide more seamless and integrated support. Schools that embrace inclusion are improving the way they meet all students' needs within the context of the general education setting through community building and differentiation, thereby giving students access to a rich social environment and the academic core curriculum.

WHAT DO I NEED TO KNOW ABOUT THE INDIVIDUALIZED EDUCATION PROGRAM?

Every student who receives special education services must have an IEP. A student who has an IEP has already been tested and observed, and a team has determined that the student has a disability. An IEP is a legal plan written by a team of professionals that documents the learning priorities for the school year (Huefner, 2000). This team includes the parent, the student (when appropriate), the general education teacher, the special education teacher, a representative of the school district, and other professionals whose expertise is needed (e.g., psychologist, SLP, OT, PT). When writing this document, the team comes together annually to determine and document the student's unique needs and goals regarding his or her participation in the general school curriculum for the upcoming school year. According to the U.S. Department of Education (2004), every IEP must legally include the following information:

- Present levels of performance—this states how a student is performing across all subject areas

- Measurable goals and objectives—this indicates the annual goals for a student across subject areas

- Special education and related services—this is the type, level, and amount of service that will be provided by special education staff

- The extent of participation with children without disabilities—the IEP must note how much time a student spends with general education peers

- A statement of how the child's progress will be measured—the team needs to describe how often and how a student's progress will be measured

- Modifications—the student's modifications or adaptations must be listed

- Participation in statewide tests—the IEP indicates whether the student will participate in statewide tests and, if so, what modifications will be provided

- Locations of services to be provided—this explains the amount of time students will receive services and the location (e.g., general education classroom)

- Statement of transition services—each student who is at least 16 years of age must have a statement of preparation for adult life

The role of the SLP in the IEP process is to help construct the present level of performance related to communication, language, and swallowing in the school environment, and to help write goals relevant to those needs. In addition, SLPs must suggest the number of minutes required to reach those goals and specify the location of services. Most inclusive related service providers figure out how to make skills fit seamlessly into the student's day and integrate the needed skills into the larger educational

Table 3.2. Examples of inclusive goals with speech-language skills embedded

Skill	Inclusive goal
Phonological sound production	Given a repeated chant during morning meeting that uses the /s/ sound, a visual model of the s, and a classroom of peers modeling the sound, Gavin will articulate the /s/ sound audibly in three out of five repeated trials.
Voice intonation	Given a community builder that requires students to ask questions, Sue will ask questions to a peer with appropriate intonation (pitch rise and respiration at the conclusion of each question) in four out of five trials.
Conversation initiation	Given lunch tables arranged by interest topics and 5 minutes of preteaching about question starters (i.e., What level are you on in Minecraft?), Caleb will initiate a conversation with a peer four out of five lunch periods a week.
Turn taking	During small-group science lab discussion using a talking object (i.e., a Koosh ball), Jay-quon will delay speaking until he is handed the Koosh ball to share on eight out of eight repeated opportunities.
Jaw position and muscle memory for speech production	Given a large piece of gum (e.g., Hubba Bubba) during large-group lecture time, Katie will chew the gum for 15-minute increments on both right and left sides to increase jaw strength and symmetrical stability for speech production.

Table 3.3. Communicating with families about inclusive services

Where will the services take place?	The services are now brought to the student, instead of having the student leave the classroom to receive services.
Will that be embarrassing for my child?	Services are not delivered at the back table in an inclusive classroom for all other students to see. Instead, each student's therapy goals are infused into the school day in a natural way.
Why will the services be delivered inclusively?	Educators are finding that students who have uninterrupted access to the general education classroom perform better overall. Federal laws have prioritized inclusive service delivery over pull-out services, as students tend to perform better when all of the therapy services are worked into the school day. Many students find leaving for therapy to be stigmatizing, and they feel an impact socially and emotionally. Skills taught in therapy settings often do not generalize to natural contexts; therefore, teaching them in a natural context the first time helps students to be able to apply the new skills.
So does that mean my child is receiving less service?	I will be working with the teacher to help to infuse all of the needed skills in the classroom, so it is likely that your child will be receiving even more services and support.

goals in the rest of the document. Examples of inclusive speech-language-pathology-infused goals are included in Table 3.2.

WHAT DO I COMMUNICATE TO FAMILIES ABOUT INCLUSIVE SERVICES?

For some families, inclusive service provision will be a new concept. School professionals may have been extolling the virtues of individual therapy to them for years. How can an SLP communicate the virtues of inclusive schooling? Table 3.3 gives ideas of what to tell families about inclusive services.

COMMONLY ASKED QUESTIONS ABOUT INCLUSIVE EDUCATION

Q. Is inclusive education really best for a particular student?

A. This question is common to teachers and SLPs alike. Research has consistently shown that the inclusive environment is better educationally and socially for students with disabilities. Our job is to figure out how to make the general education environment suitable to the student's needs.

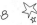

Q. How do I meet the number of minutes for SLP services on the IEPs unless I pull students out?

A. Services can be carried out in many ways. The law suggests that services are portable and should be brought to the student. Therefore, your time could be spent pushing in to the general education classroom, running a center, or recommending ideas to the other educators on how to carry out the specific skills while they teach. Your time could be spent modifying or adapting the material so the student can be successful in the general education classroom and throughout the school day.

Q. I have so many students on my workload, how can I get to them all inclusively?

A. One thing that has become clear in the law is that staff convenience is not a reason to pull students. Therefore, you might determine which students need direct support, which students can receive consult services, and for which students you will stop by to monitor progress. Then, arrange your schedule to match those needs. Instead of thinking about your workload as static and unchanging (e.g., 11:30–11:45, Zack receives oral motor stimulation in the speech and language room), you begin to think of appropriate times to provide such services, and generally problem solve across Zack's day.

Q. Is inclusion really the law?

A. IDEA 2004 does not use the term *inclusion*. Nonetheless, the law stipulates that all students must be placed in the LRE. The first consideration must be the general education setting, and schools must prove that they have attempted to teach all children in the general education setting with appropriate supplementary aids and services before considering placement in more restrictive settings.

CONCLUSION

Schools today are becoming increasingly inclusive. Therefore, SLPs working in inclusive settings need to understand the rationale for inclusive schooling, the history of inclusive schooling, major concepts in inclusive schooling, indicators of inclusion, and the concept of the IEP as a framework to most fully support students in inclusive settings. You will not be expected to do this alone; you will be part of an educational team. The next chapter focuses on how you as an SLP fit into a collaborative team that will work to educate all students.

NOTES

_____

_____

_____

_____

_____

_____

_____

_____

_____

_____

_____

_____

_____

_____

_____

_____

_____

_____

_____

_____

_____

_____

_____

_____

_____

4

Collaborating with Others

Working within a Team

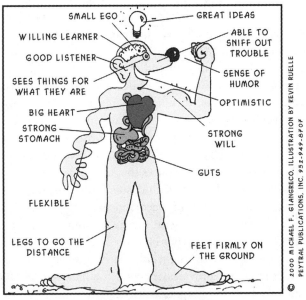

ANATOMY OF AN
EFFECTIVE TEAM MEMBER

"When I was doing pull-out service delivery, it was harder to collaborate with teachers. It was harder to spend the time sitting down and showing them what I am doing with the kids. And it's easier this way, when I provide collaborative services, because I think sometimes teachers think . . . that we're doing something completely different in our room and we have this little magical dust! I think now the teachers are kind of learning 'oh okay well I can do that' and then they are more likely to want to work together as a team to meet both the academic and therapy goals. I think that it is better for the kids, and that's the most important thing!"

—Ella (SLP)

"We've each been invited to this present moment by design. Our lives are joined together like the tiles of a mosaic; none of us contributes the whole of the picture, but each of us is necessary for its completion."

—Casey & Vanceburg (1996, p. 138)

All students in a classroom community can benefit from a team of professionals working together, which includes therapists, teachers, and paraprofessionals working together in ways that promote meaningful learning and a sense of belonging for all students. This collaboration between professionals on educating students with disabilities is a fundamental aspect of the federal IDEA 2004 legislation (PL 108-446, §614[d][1][B]; §636[a][1]; §652[b][1]; §653[b]; §654[a][1][C]). In an inclusive classroom, the professionals are like tiles of a mosaic. Each person is an important contributor to the larger picture. In today's inclusive classrooms, it is quite common for general education teachers and special education teachers to work alongside therapists and paraprofessionals.

This chapter provides information and tools that will enable SLPs to engage in effective collaboration. To achieve this, the available resources are maximized to ensure all students' participation, content learning, and meeting of IEP goals. In some cases, however, teachers, therapists, and paraprofessionals work in isolation in the planning or implementation stages. A common problem that arises from this is that therapists, who may have unclear roles in the classroom, feel devalued and like glorified teaching assistants when they provide push-in services that are not meaningfully planned. Purposeful planning is needed to align curriculum standards, learning strategies, teaching strategies, and therapy interventions to meet students' IEP goals.

This chapter will help you to see your role as a member of the larger educational team and to address the roles and responsibilities of each team member. We propose general ways to communicate with the whole teaching team, outline co-teaching or co-supporting structures, and provide strategies for handling conflict. Finally, we address commonly asked questions about collaboration.

ROLES AND RESPONSIBILITIES

Roles and responsibilities of school professionals vary among schools, districts, and even states. Nonetheless, despite these variations, there are generally accepted roles and responsibilities that hold true from school to school. The next subsections provide some general guidelines for how school personnel can work effectively as a team to meet the needs of all students together.

Speech-Language Pathologists

SLPs help students with all of the skills required to communicate effectively. These skills include all issues related to language, the voice and sound production, articulation, swallowing, fluency, and cognition. Some students who work with SLPs have issues with stuttering. Others work on understanding and producing language. Some students need support with executive functioning, memory, problem solving, and other cognition elements. The SLP brings a unique expertise that contributes greatly to educational teams. In schools, SLPs collaborate with teaching teams to support classroom activities and effective communication.

Special Educators

A special educator is partly responsible for designing each student's IEP. Each year, a team of teachers and parents determines each student's goals and objectives and the appropriate special education services. The special education teacher helps to ensure that the goals and objectives on each student's IEP are met. In collaboration with general education teachers, therapists, and other support staff, the special education teacher is responsible for helping to differentiate curricula and instruction, and provides and recommends modifications and adaptations that would be appropriate for each student. Special education teachers are also responsible for solving problems that arise in the classroom, evaluating each student's services, and communicating student progress to the team.

General Educators

A general educator can be expected to educate the students in his or her class. A general educator plans lessons, teaches those lessons, and assesses each student's skill. A general educator is responsible not only for each student with an IEP but also for all of the students who do not have disabilities. Typically, a general educator is considered the content expert for the particular grade level being taught.

The Family

Family members are undoubtedly the most important people in a child's life. With the reauthorization of IDEA 2004, parents or legal guardians became equal members of students' IEP teams. Parents or guardians are expected to be active members of their children's education teams, because they know their children better than anyone else. Therapists, teachers, and paraprofessionals can help parents play active roles by communicating all that happens in the school setting and, further, by listening closely to the wishes and concerns of family members.

Physical Therapists

Physical therapy is another related service and is provided by a qualified and licensed PT. PTs address areas such as gross motor development skills, orthopedic concerns, mobility, adaptive equipment, positioning needs, and other functional skills that may interfere with students' educational performance. Similar to an SLP, a PT either works with individual students or leads small groups. PTs also consult with teachers, other therapists, and paraprofessionals. Specific types of therapies include practice walking up and down stairs safely, body stretching for students who use a wheelchair, supporting access to school environments, or help performing other physical activities.

Physical Therapy Assistants

Some PTs have assistants who are responsible for carrying out therapy plans, supporting in classrooms and the school environment, keeping track of data for the IEP goals, and supporting self-care needs. These assistants work under the direction of certified PTs.

Occupational Therapists

For a student who works with an OT, the student's disability necessitates support in daily life skills or functioning throughout the school day. The therapist may evaluate the student's needs, provide therapy, modify classroom equipment, restructure environmental conditions, and generally help the student participate as fully as possible in school experiences and activities. A therapist may work with children individually or lead small groups. Therapists also may consult with teachers and paraprofessionals to help students meet their goals within the context of general education settings. Specific types of therapies may include help with handwriting or computer work, fostering social play, and teaching life skills such as getting dressed or eating with utensils. The difference between the role of OT and PT can be confusing; in general, OTs work more with fine motor skills and PTs work more with gross motor skills.

Occupational Therapy Assistants

Some OTs have assistants who are responsible for carrying out therapy plans, supporting in classrooms and the school environment, keeping track of data for the IEP goals, and supporting self-care needs. These assistants work under the direction of certified OTs.

School Psychologists

The goals of school psychologists are to "help children and youth succeed academically, socially, and emotionally" (National Association of School Psychologists [NASP], 2000). School psychologists work closely with teaching teams to create healthy and safe learning environments and to strengthen connections between each student's home and school. Psychologists assess students and are often involved in standardized testing to determine whether a student qualifies as having a disability. Psychologists also work directly with others on teaching teams by helping to problem-solve and, at times, provide direct support services to students.

School Social Workers

Like psychologists, school social workers help provide links connecting each student's home, school, and community. The services provided by social workers are intended to help enable students and families to overcome problems that may impede learning. School social workers provide individual and group counseling, consult with teachers, and teach or encourage social skills. They collaborate with community agencies and provide service coordination for students who require many different agencies or services.

Vision Teachers

Vision teachers support students who have VIs or blindness. Vision teachers typically work with classroom teachers to make modifications and adaptations to the curricula. They also help provide needed equipment (e.g., magnifiers and computer equipment) and needed materials (e.g., worksheets in braille).

Audiologists

Audiologists typically work with students who have hearing impairments, providing amplification systems and sign language interpreters for students who are deaf.

Paraprofessionals

Paraprofessionals are expected to perform many different tasks. Supporting students academically, socially, and behaviorally in the school community is essential. Paraprofessionals review and reinforce instruction, under the direction of special education teachers or general education teachers. They might lead a station lesson, read aloud, or team-teach with other educators. Paraprofessionals might also assist the teachers in daily paperwork of the classroom. Paraprofessionals are vital in facilitating social interactions between students.

HOW DO ALL THESE PEOPLE WORK TOGETHER?

"The games I used to use in my therapy room for speech production and communication are now part of the general education classroom. Several of the teachers I work with now use these games as a center in their rooms. One uses several of the communication games for

choice time with the students. Now, when I run a center . . . it is clear that these games are benefiting everyone as they all work on skill development at different levels."

—Rose (SLP)

Every school differs, but one thing is certain: all the adults on a teaching team must work together for the purpose of promoting student growth. One example of effective collaboration involves a seventh-grade team.

· · · · · · · · · ·

This team involves all of the staff members who support Adam, a student with autism, a visual impairment, and sensory needs. The core team of people supporting Adam in English class includes the general education teacher, the SLP, the OT, the vision teacher, the special education teacher, and a paraprofessional. This team meets monthly to discuss Adam's support in English class. Every week, the vision teacher and the English teacher meet with the paraprofessional to create enlarged materials for upcoming units of study. In addition, the special education teacher and the English teacher plan lessons together with Adam in mind so that each lesson is designed to meet his needs. For example, they planned a unit using a book from the Harry Potter series. In addition to having the paraprofessional enlarge the text in the packet of information, the teacher decided to have the entire class listen to an audio version of the book instead of reading silently. The OT set up a box of sensory tools with fidgets, pencil grips, a choice of writing utensils, an AlphaSmart keyboard, and gum. The OT joins the meeting to problem-solve sensory-related issues in English class. The SLP meets with the team to provide indirect services related to Adam's language pragmatic development. He is working on social aspects of communication throughout his school day, and the team purposefully embeds social interactions during learning experiences. The SLP suggests that the class have stopping points every 10 minutes during the audio book to allow students to engage in a "walk and talk" regarding comprehension questions of the story. This ensures Adam's social communication goals are embedded during English class. This plan outlines the anticipated type and level of support that Adam needs during each activity.

· · · · · · · · · ·

Your team can fill out the grid in Figure 4.1 to help determine the roles and responsibilities of all of your teammates. Many teams have found it useful to determine who has primary, secondary, and shared responsibilities for each of the necessary tasks in inclusive classrooms. Then together, answer the questions that follow, to help make decisions about whether any roles should be changed or shared.

GUIDING QUESTIONS FOR TEAMS TO DISCUSS

Getting to know your teammates on a personal level is necessary for real and true collaboration to occur. Some questions that will help you as you sit down with teachers,

Determining Roles and Responsibilities Among Team Members

Directions: Read through the following common roles and responsibilities. Determine which team member should take on each of the roles and responsibilities:

P = Primary responsibility   S = Secondary responsibility

Sh = Shared responsibility   I = Input in the decision making

Major role or responsibility	Classroom teacher	Special education teacher	Speech-language pathologist	Paraprofessional
Developing student objectives				
Designing differentiated curriculum				
Creating student-specific modifications and adaptations				
Creating classroom materials				
Co-teaching curriculum				
Providing one-to-one instruction				
Teaching the whole class of students				
Leading small groups				
Monitoring student progress				
Examining student work to determine next steps				
Assessing and assigning grades				
Communicating with parents				
Consulting with related service personnel				
Participating in IEP meetings				

Figure 4.1. Determining Roles and Responsibilities Among Team Members form.   *(continued)*

Adapted by permission from Causton-Theoharis, J. (2003). *Increasing interactions between students with disabilities and their peers via paraprofessional training* (Unpublished doctoral dissertation). University of Wisconsin–Madison. Reprinted from Causton, J., & Theoharis, G. (2014). *The principal's handbook for leading inclusive schools* (pp. 80–81). Baltimore, MD: Paul H. Brookes Publishing Co.

In *The Speech-Language Pathologist's Handbook for Inclusive School Practices* by Julie Causton and Chelsea P. Tracy-Bronson (2014, Paul H. Brookes Publishing Co., Inc.)

Figure 4.1. *(continued)* (page 2 of 2)

Disciplining students				
Writing in communication notebooks				
Providing community-based programming				

Major role or responsibility	Classroom teacher	Special education teacher	Speech-language pathologist	Paraprofessional
Developing peer supports				
Scheduling common planning time				
Participating in regularly scheduled team planning meetings				
Facilitating meetings				
Communicating information from meetings to other team members				
Other				

When you have finished determining roles and responsibilities for each of the team members, ask yourselves the following questions:

1. Could any of these roles and responsibilities be shared or changed?

2. Does anyone feel uncomfortable with any of the roles as outlined?

3. Does anyone believe he or she needs more information or training to perform the above-mentioned responsibilities?

4. What messages are sent to students, parents, and others about the way adults work together as a team in this classroom through the division of responsibilities?

5. What changes need to be made?

Adapted by permission from Causton-Theoharis, J. (2003). *Increasing interactions between students with disabilities and their peers via paraprofessional training* (Unpublished doctoral dissertation). University of Wisconsin–Madison. Reprinted from Causton, J., & Theoharis, G. (2014). *The principal's handbook for leading inclusive schools* (pp. 80–81). Baltimore, MD: Paul H. Brookes Publishing Co.

In *The Speech-Language Pathologist's Handbook for Inclusive School Practices* by Julie Causton and Chelsea P. Tracy-Bronson (2014, Paul H. Brookes Publishing Co., Inc.)

other therapists, or paraprofessionals are listed in this section. You may consider this list as some simple suggestions, or you may decide to go through each question with your team.

Work Styles

- Are you a morning or afternoon person?
- How direct are you?
- Do you like to do several things at once, or do you prefer doing one thing at a time?
- How do you prefer to give feedback to others on the team?
- What do you consider your strengths and weaknesses when working in a team situation?

Philosophy

- The goal of therapy provision should occur . . .
- To me, *normalcy* means . . .
- It's important to consider functioning level versus social relationships because . . .
- To me, *advanced planning* means . . .
- All kids learn best when . . .
- In general, I think the best way to deal with challenging behavior is . . .
- In general, I think it is important to increase student independence by . . .
- I think our team relationship needs to be . . .

Logistics

- How should we communicate about students' history and progress?
- How should we communicate about our roles and responsibilities?
- How and when should we communicate about lessons and modifications?
- If I do not know an answer in class, should I direct the student to you?
- Do we meet often enough? If not, when should we meet?
- How do we communicate with the families? What is each person's role in this?
- Are there other logistical concerns?

Questions for the Family

- How would you like to communicate about your child's progress?
- If we are using a communication notebook or e-mail, how often would you like to hear from the school?
- Are there things you are especially interested in hearing about?

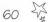

After having personal discussions using these questions as a guide, teams are better able to negotiate the logistical and philosophical components of teamwork, allowing team members to feel more comfortable in knowing the roles and expectations within the classroom setting. The next section describes some co-teaching and co-supporting arrangements that should give further clarity to the collaborative work of educational professionals in the classroom.

CO-SUPPORTING ARRANGEMENTS

Because SLPs generally do not introduce or teach new academic content, we have adapted some co-teaching arrangements from Friend and Reising (1993) and have created co-supporting arrangements. Schraeder (2013) called these arrangements complementary teaching and team teaching.

One Teach, One Observe

While the teacher is teaching, you might observe and take progress-monitoring data on student performance. You also could collect information on the students' skills as they relate to speech and language therapy skills and the next steps. You might observe the effectiveness of a specific assistive technology, new positioning arrangements, or other type of support.

One Teach, One Support

While the teacher is instructing in the large group, you might provide support to students in the class. You could help students choose which type of writing paper or tools fit their needs. You also could write or draw examples on the chalkboard. Taking visual notes that include diagrams, pictures, and labels is a useful strategy when one educator is teaching. If a student whom you support has significant needs (e.g., a seizure disorder or medical needs that require proximity), you will want to remain close to the student. However, for the most part, you should help all students even though you are providing services to specific students.

Station Facilitation

An SLP can run a small group or a station. It is important, however, for SLPs to first plan this station in concert with a general education or special education teacher so that both academic content and therapy skills are present. Co-planning and co-supporting the implementation of stations in the classroom allows students with disabilities to continue having access to general education curriculum, work on therapy goals, and continue to be educated in the LRE alongside peers.

Co-Support

Another common type of support is called co-support. While the teacher is leading the large group, you can ask clarifying questions or provide examples. Table 4.1 shows

Table 4.1. Ideas for providing engaged therapy co-support

If the teacher is doing this	You can be doing this
Lecturing	Providing visual notes simultaneously to allow students to see what they are listening to. Creating graphic organizers that allow students to remember key words and phrases. Providing sentence starters.
Giving directions	Writing the directions on the board so all students have a place to look for the visual cues. Providing to-do lists or individual agendas for students with reminders or cues for positioning.
Providing large-group instruction	Collecting data, problem solving, improving environmental factors (e.g., lighting), or making modifications for an upcoming lesson
Giving a test	Reading the test to students who prefer to have the test read to them. Before the test, making sure the student is well positioned, lighting is right, and test is modified to support the student's learning strengths (e.g., enlarged font or one problem per page).
Facilitating stations or small groups	Also facilitating stations or groups
Teaching a new concept	Providing visuals or models to enhance the whole group's understanding. Creating a multisensory approach to the content to increase the learning for all.
Reteaching or preteaching with a small group	Monitoring the large group as the students work independently. Thinking about body positioning and learning environment for all students.

Source: Murawski and Dieker (2004).

some types of co-support you might provide in different situations, as suggested by Murawski and Dieker (2004).

Therapy Plan at a Glance

The Therapy Plan at a Glance is useful for SLPs to communicate the priority skills for a supported student, as well as the useful materials and verbal prompts used to help each student practice the skill within the context of an inclusive classroom. One SLP we know fills out a Therapy Plan at a Glance for every student on her caseload, photocopies them, and dispenses them to all educational team members, special area teachers, and substitutes who work with the student. See Figure 4.2 for an example. See Figure 4.3 for a Program Planning Matrix that you can use.

WHAT IF CONFLICT ARISES?

"It wasn't adjusting my therapy services that proved to be difficult. That took a little bit of time to change how I planned for sessions each week because now I was doing it with the others on the team, and it was rewarding. But, really the most challenging thing was working in the same physical space as teachers who taught very differently, talked to kids differently ... there was one who just had an opposite disposition from me, and that took a while to get used to."

—Shelby (SLP)

Ideal team functioning is like a well-oiled machine in which each cog runs continually and smoothly, each harmoniously performing an individual function for the good

Dear Educational Team,

Chloe is working on the following speech and language skills (see the left-hand side). It would be beneficial to provide him or her with as many opportunities with these activities as possible (see the right-hand side).

Skills	Activities
Swallowing	Drinking, sucking on a straw, chewing gum, small snack eating (i.e., Cheerios)
Producing the /l/ sound	Songs, chants, rhymes with the repeated /l/ sound.
Voice volume	Walk-talks, presenting to peers, partner work, opportunities to socialize

I use the following materials and prompts to help support these skills within your classroom. Let's try to reinforce these new skills throughout the day.

Swallowing	Materials with activity	Prompts
Producing the /l/ sound	Feeding aids (adapted spoon)	Just present student with the modified cup and spoon when needed
Voice volume (for student who whispers when talking)	Modified cup Picture support with the ABC chart Megaphone Audio recorder	"Tongue on top teeth." "Open your mouth." "Can they hear you in the back of the room?" "Can you hear yourself?" "Volume level 5."

Additional tips and tricks:

I will drop off the audio recorder; Chloe likes to play it back when she reads. This could be a center for all during practice for Readers Theater. I will also drop off the feeding aids (cup and spoon).

For the /l/ sound production, please provide as many practice trials during the day that naturally occur. She becomes embarrassed if it seems like someone is correcting her speech, so just provide opportunities for practice and help with data collection (on the sheets provided). Also, be sure to clearly model /l/ sound production during phonics instruction. It is most helpful if these skills are seamlessly built in and not made obvious to her or her peers.

Please allow Chloe to have water throughout the day; this helps with both swallowing and drooling. Additionally, she needs permission to chew gum during the day. I have a story that explains gum chewing to the students; I am happy to come and read it if you would like. This helps students understand Chloe's swallowing and drooling issues and helps students know how to best support her. I asked Chloe and her parents, and she would like the book read to her classmates.

Please contact me. I am always available for problem solving.

Debbie Smith

Figure 4.2. Speech-Language Pathology Therapy Plan at a Glance example.

Program Planning Matrix

Student: _____

Class: _____   Date: _____

Class Schedule

Individualized education program goals							

Key: X = instruction provided; O = classroom participation plans with general adaptations required;
• = general adaptations plan and weekly plan for specific adaptations required

Figure 4.3. Program Planning Matrix.

Adapted by permission from Janney, R., & Snell, M.E. (2004). *Teachers' guides to inclusive practices: Modifying schoolwork* (2nd ed., p. 131). Baltimore, MD: Paul H. Brookes Publishing Co. Reprinted in Causton, J., & Tracy-Bronson, C.P. (2014). *The occupational therapist's handbook for inclusive school practices*. Baltimore, MD: Paul H. Brookes Publishing Co.

In *The Speech-Language Pathologist's Handbook for Inclusive School Practices* by Julie Causton and Chelsea P. Tracy-Bronson (2014, Paul H. Brookes Publishing Co., Inc.)

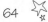

of the entire machine. However, team functioning does not always feel this smooth. Conflicts among adults do arise.

The Bonner Foundation, a nonprofit education organization, has suggested eight steps for conflict resolution. *Conflict* is defined as "a mental or physical disagreement in which people's values or needs are in opposition to each other or they think that they are opposed" (Bonner Foundation, 2008). The Bonner Foundation's suggestions for handling conflicts are listed here, along with our related suggestions:

1. "Identify positions ('what are they saying') of each side of the people in conflict." Write down your perspective and the other person's perspective.

2. "Learn more about true needs and desires behind each side." Write down your beliefs about the other person's needs and desires. Write down your own needs and desires.

3. "Ask clarifying questions for more information." Ask the other person, "Why do you feel the way you do?" "What do you think you need in this situation?" Reframe the problem into a question.

4. "Brainstorm possible solutions." Without judging the ideas, write down as many ideas as you can.

5. "Discuss how each solution would affect each side, and figure out possible compromises." Talk through each of the potential solutions. Discuss which ones would work and which ones would not work, from your perspective and from the other person's perspective. Generate more ideas, if necessary.

6. "Agree on a solution." Determine which solution would work the best for both of you. Write out a plan for carrying out the solution and determine how long you plan to implement the solution.

7. "Implement solutions." Give your idea a try for the determined amount of time.

8. "Reevaluate solutions, if necessary." Come back together to discuss the solution and what is working or not working about this solution. Continue the process as necessary.

MAKING THE TIME TO COMMUNICATE

One of the most common problems SLPs mention involves not having enough time to communicate or collaborate with the teachers with whom they work. When they do have or find the time, some find that the meetings are not efficient or well-planned. Many teams utilize team meeting minutes (see Figure 4.4) as a way to make meetings more effective. For teams that struggle to find meeting times, different school teams have solved this problem by using several strategies. Each strategy is described in the following list. Examine each strategy and see whether it will help your team to

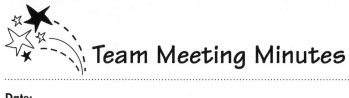

Team Meeting Minutes

Date: _____

Team members present and assigned roles: **Team members absent:**

Facilitator:

Recorder:

Timekeeper:

Consensus builder:

Observer:

Today's agenda items	I - Information D - Discussion R - Requires decision	Presenter	Time guidelines
1.			
2.			
3.			
4.			
5.			
6.			

Items discussed:

(continued)

Figure 4.4. Team Meeting Minutes form.

From Causton, J., & Theoharis, G. (2014). *The principal's handbook for leading inclusive schools* (pp. 70–71). Baltimore, MD: Paul H. Brookes Publishing Co., Inc.; reprinted by permission.

In *The Speech-Language Pathologist's Handbook for Inclusive School Practices* by Julie Causton and Chelsea P. Tracy-Bronson (2014, Paul H. Brookes Publishing Co., Inc.)

Figure 4.4. *(continued)*   (page 2 of 2)

Task delegated, time lines, follow-up:

Activity	Person responsible	Time line

Agenda items for next meeting:

1.

2.

3.

4.

5.

6.

Next meeting date: _____

From Causton, J., & Theoharis, G. (2014). *The principal's handbook for leading inclusive schools* (pp. 70–71). Baltimore, MD: Paul H. Brookes Publishing Co., Inc.; reprinted by permission.

In *The Speech-Language Pathologist's Handbook for Inclusive School Practices* by Julie Causton and Chelsea P. Tracy-Bronson (2014, Paul H. Brookes Publishing Co., Inc.)

communicate more regularly and more effectively. The following strategies have been successfully used to carve out more meeting time:

- *Video or independent work time*—Create a weekly meeting time during which students are expected to watch instructional videos or to work independently for 15 minutes. Allow them to watch or work independently while the team meets.

- *Use a parent volunteer*—As a parent volunteer reads a book to the students or leads a review game, meet together for 15 minutes.

- *Use another teacher team*—Put two classrooms together for a half hour each week for a certain portion of the curriculum or community-building activities. One teaching team supervises the students while the other team meets. The teams then switch.

- *Meet during specials time*—Ask the specials teachers whether their schedule has an extra 15 minutes during any one day. Use that time to meet together.

- *Meet before or after school*—Take 15 minutes before or after school to have a "sacred" meeting time for teaching teams.

If you simply cannot use any of these strategies to elicit more face-to-face meeting times, some teams have come up with alternatives to meeting face-to-face.

- *Communication notebook*—Establish a notebook that all members of the team read and respond to each day. Team members can write questions in the notebook and obtain responses. Notebooks also can be used to discuss schedules or student-specific information.

- *E-mail*—E-mail can be substituted for the communication notebook; team members can contact each other with questions, comments, or schedule changes.

- *Mailbox*—Use a mailbox in the classroom for each staff member. Direct all notes or general information to that place.

- *Proofread*—As notes are written that go home to the students' parents, have the teaching team proofread each of the notes. This way, not only are the notes proofread, but everyone receives all of the necessary information.

- *Lesson plan sharing*—Keep lesson plans out and accessible to all members of the team. Use the notes to communicate about upcoming content. Ask the person who writes the plans to delineate each team member's role for each lesson. The educational team might also keep lesson plans electronically on a shared space for ease of collaboration.

COMMONLY ASKED QUESTIONS ABOUT COLLABORATION

Q. I am not sure what I am supposed to be doing when I provide push-in services. We (the general education teacher and I) have never co-designed or collaborated to plan lessons, so mostly I just sit and support two students who receive speech-language pathology as part of their IEP goals. What should I do?

A. Set up a time to meet with the general education teacher. Ask questions such as, "How can we both have useful roles during science, while meeting Zack and Priscilla's therapy goals?" "When you are giving whole-class instructions, how can I support you?" "How can you integrate Zack's therapy goals during the rest of the day?" These conversations that merge academic learning experiences with therapy interventions are crucial in ensuring that IEP goals are generalized throughout the day.

Q. I have read about common co-teaching and co-supporting arrangements, but we do not use any of them at my school; instead, I just sit and support or walk around and support. How can I suggest that we use these strategies?

A. Show your teaching partner the different arrangements. Begin a conversation asking whether the arrangements might be useful to your team. Sketch a diagram that shows what each of the co-teaching arrangements look like: This helps others envision teaching arrangement possibilities. Let the teachers know that you are willing to have a meaningful co-supporting role in their inclusive classroom.

Q. What if I feel uncomfortable with a role I have been assigned?

A. Communicate your concerns to your teaching team. The role might not have to be changed; it could be shared. If you believe you are being asked to do something outside the scope of your job, talk to the teaching team first and then to your principal or director of special education.

CONCLUSION

Working as a team member and within a school setting can be challenging, but it also can be rewarding. Understanding each team member's roles, including your own, can bring clarity to your work. Learning more information about each of your teammates is essential to building trust within your team. Further, using common co-teaching and co-supporting arrangements can clarify specific roles and responsibilities within the classroom. Communication is key; the more effectively you communicate and solve conflicts as you work together, the better your team will function, enabling you to deliver more seamless support to students. Chapter 5 focuses on how to rethink students in terms of their strengths, gifts, and talents so that they can reach their full academic potential.

NOTES

_____

_____

_____

_____

_____

_____

_____

_____

_____

_____

_____

_____

_____

_____

_____

_____

_____

_____

_____

_____

_____

_____

_____

_____

5

Rethinking Students

Presuming Competence

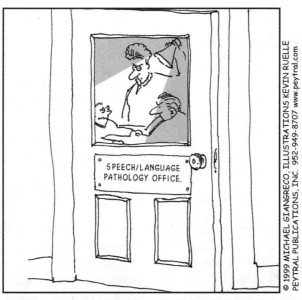

© 1999 MICHAEL GIANGRECO. ILLUSTRATIONS KEVIN RUELLE
PEYTRAL PUBLICATIONS, INC. 952-949-8707 www.peytral.com

SPEECH/LANGUAGE
PATHOLOGY OFFICE.

"WE HAVE WAYS OF MAKING YOU TALK!"

"I think the field of rehabilitation is to people with disabilities what the diet industry is to women. We live in a society that idolizes a full and completely artificial conception of bodily perfection. This view of the 'normal' body tyrannizes most, if not all, women so that far too many women in our culture grow up believing that their bodies are inadequate in some way. The issue here is that I want professionals to think about the whole parallel between dieting and rehabilitation. That's why I always tell people with disabilities, 'Never do physical therapy with a therapist who is on a diet!' If she hates her own body, she'll inevitably do harm to yours!"

—Norman Kunc (Giangreco, 1996/2004, p. 36)

"When I approach a child, [s]he inspires in me two sentiments: tenderness for what [s]he is, and respect for what [s]he may become."

—Louis Pasteur (Institut Pasteur, n.d.)

This chapter introduces the concept of *rethinking students*. Rethinking a student entails getting to know about the student and then reflecting on how you see, treat, provide services to, and work with him or her. First, we discuss how to describe students to others through student strengths and multiple intelligences. Then, we describe the concept of presumption of competence and using age-appropriate and person-first language. Please see Table 5.1 for examples of person-first language (Snow, 2008).

STUDENT DESCRIPTIONS

Shawntell Strully is a 22-year-old who lives in her own home with roommates, attends classes at Colorado State University, volunteers on campus, travels during spring break, gets around in her own car, has her own interests, likes and desires, has a boyfriend, and speaks out on issues of concern to her.

Shawntell Strully is 22 years old, is severely/profoundly mentally retarded, is hearing impaired, visually impaired, has cerebral palsy, has a seizure disorder, does not chew her food (and sometimes chokes), is not toilet trained, has no verbal communication, has no reliable communication system, and has a developmental age of 17–24 months.

(Strully & Strully, 1996, pp. 144–145)

These two radically different descriptions of Shawntell come from two different groups of people. The first description comes from her parents. The second comes from her teachers and other school support personnel. Although not all educational professionals would describe Shawntell in these ways, this is how her team described her. It is surprising to compare these statements side by side. The stark contrast raises the question of how the same person can be described in such disparate ways.

The principal reason for these radically different descriptions is that each group of people looks for different things and approaches Shawntell from a different perspective. Shawntell's parents know her deeply. They have spent a great deal of time

Table 5.1. Examples of person-first language

Say	Instead of	Because
People with disabilities	The disabled or handicapped	Place emphasis on the person.
People without disabilities	Normal/healthy/typical	The nonpreferred terms assume the opposite for students with disabilities (e.g., abnormal, unhealthy, atypical).
Ella, the fourth-grade student	Ella, the student with Down syndrome	Omit the label whenever possible; it is most often not relevant.
Communicates with her eyes/device, and so forth	Is nonverbal	Focus on strengths.
Uses a wheelchair	Is confined to a wheelchair	Use possessive language to refer to assistive technologies; the nonpreferred language implies the person is "stuck."
Accessible parking spot	Handicapped parking spot	Accurate representation
Beth has autism.	Beth is autistic.	Emphasize that disability is one attribute—not a defining characteristic.
Gail has a learning disability.	Gail is learning disabled.	Emphasize that disability is one attribute—not a defining characteristic.
Jeff has a cognitive disability.	Jeff is retarded.	Emphasize that disability is one attribute—not a defining characteristic; also, *cognitive disability* is a preferred term.
Ben receives special education services.	Ben is in special education.	Special education is a service, not a place.
The student who is blind	The blind student	Place the person before the disability.
Denis writes using the computer.	Denis cannot write with a pencil.	Focus on strengths.
Needs a magnifier, laptop, or cane	Problems with vision; cannot write or walk	Focus on needs, not problems.

Source: Snow (2008).

with her, know her intimately, and understand her as a person who has wide interests and capabilities. Their description of her cites her interests, gifts, and talents. Conversely, the description generated by Shawntell's educational team reflects a more distant understanding of her; it is a cold, clinical account that focuses exclusively on her impairments.

As an SLP working with students with disabilities, you will hear impairment-driven descriptions of students, and, thus, you will need to work to understand these students through their strengths, gifts, and talents. You may read a student's IEP, and it might abound with terms such as *mental age of 2, phobic,* or *aggressive.* Reading those descriptors, you will need to realize that you are getting only one perspective on the student. Get to know the student yourself, develop an authentic relationship, and work to learn about what he or she can do. Ideally, your descriptions of a student would look much closer to the parents' perspective on Shawntell than that of the teachers.

BEGIN WITH STRENGTHS

We were talking to Joe and asked him to describe Mary, a student who receives related services. He described Mary as autistic, loud, sensitive, a runner, sometimes sweet, a mover, and nonverbal. These descriptions speak to Joe's own beliefs about the student. On a piece of paper, write down the first 10 descriptors that come to mind when you think of an individual student. Now, look over the list. Were your descriptors positive, negative, or a combination?

Your beliefs about a student will affect how you support and work with that student. For example, if you believe a student is lazy or defiant, you will approach him or her in a different way than you will if you believe that child is motivated or cooperative. You can alter your beliefs about students by spending some time rethinking them. Reframing your conceptions of students in more positive ways creates opportunities for growth.

Consider the work of educational researcher Thomas Armstrong (2000a, 2000b) on using multiple intelligence theory in the classroom. Armstrong recommended that education professionals purposefully rethink the ways they describe students. By changing their language, people will begin to change their impressions. Armstrong emphasized that all behavior is part of the human experience and that behavior is based on a multitude of influences (e.g., environment, sense of safety, and personal well-being). Armstrong has proposed that instead of considering a child learning disabled, people should see the child as *learning differently*. Table 5.2 lists further suggestions for describing students.

What would happen if all education professionals changed how they viewed and spoke about students? What if every student was viewed as a capable learner? One of the best ways to think about the students you support is to look at the child through the lens of his or her strengths. Ask yourself the following questions: "What can this student do?" "What are this person's strengths?" "How would a parent who deeply loves this student speak about him or her?" Now, return to your list and take a moment to develop a list of strengths, gifts, and interests.

During a professional development day with general educators, special educators, therapists, and paraprofessionals, Suzie did just that. First, she wrote a list of descriptors. Then, after spending some time rethinking the student, she came up with a completely different list. She had originally described the student, Brian, as "lazy, smart, sneaky, a liar, cute, cunning, and mean (at times)." After talking about viewing students differently, she got a new piece of paper. She wrote, "relaxed, intelligent, good in math, cute, needs some support with peer relationships, a great sense of humor, and a beautiful smile." Julie asked Suzie whether this still accurately described Brian. She said that the second list was a much more accurate description of him.

MULTIPLE INTELLIGENCES

There is a pervasive myth in education that some people are smart and others are not. *Intelligence, functioning level, communication level, academic potential, pragmatic*

Table 5.2. Turning lead into gold

A child who is judged to be	Can also be considered
Learning disabled	Learning differently
Hyperactive	Kinesthetic
Impulsive	Spontaneous
ADD/ADHD[a]	A bodily-kinesthetic learner
Dyslexic	A spatial learner
Aggressive	Assertive
Plodding	Thorough
Lazy	Relaxed
Immature	Late blooming
Phobic	Cautious
Scattered	Divergent
Daydreaming	Imaginative
Irritable	Sensitive
Perseverative	Persistent

From Armstrong, T. (2000a). "Table 10–1: Turning lead into gold", from IN THEIR OWN WAY by Thomas Armstrong, copyright © 1987, 2000 by Thomas Armstrong. Used by permission of Jeremy P. Tarcher, an imprint of Penguin Group (USA) LLC.
[a]ADD, attention deficit disorder; ADHD, attention-deficit/hyperactivity disorder.

skill, and *competence* are words often used to describe "smartness." In education, this belief can best be seen through the system of labeling people with disabilities. A clear example is IQ testing. Students take IQ tests, and if a student's IQ score falls below 70 and he or she has other issues with functional skills, the student receives the label of ID. Howard Gardner (1993) challenged the way psychologists and educators defined intelligences and offered a different way to look at intelligence. He used the term *multiple intelligences.*

Gardner viewed each of the multiple intelligences as a capacity that is inherent in the human brain and that is developed and expressed in social and cultural contexts. Instead of viewing intelligence as a fixed number on an aptitude test, Gardner argued that every person, regardless of disability label, is smart in different ways. All of the eight intelligences are described in Table 5.3. We have also added a column entitled "So support using," which might help you think of the students to whom you provide speech and language services. If you work with a student who prefers to learn in a certain intelligence area or who is strong in a certain area, consider some of the suggested activities and teaching styles.

PRESUME COMPETENCE

In the school setting, assumptions about students can affect their education. Take Sue Rubin, for instance.

Table 5.3. A guide to supporting through multiple intelligences

Intelligence	Which means	So support using
Verbal/linguistic intelligence	Good with words and language, written and spoken	Jokes, speeches, readings, stories, essays, the Internet, books, biographies
Logical mathematical intelligence	Preference for reasoning, numbers, and patterns	Mazes, puzzles, time lines, analogies, formulas, calculations, codes, games, probabilities
Spatial intelligence	Ability to visualize an object or to create mental images or pictures	Mosaics, drawings, illustrations, models, maps, videos, posters
Bodily kinesthetic intelligence	Knowledge or wisdom of the body and movement	Role-playing, skits, facial expressions, experiments, field trips, sports, games
Musical intelligence	Ability to recognize tonal patterns including sensitivity to rhythms or beats	Performances, songs, instruments, rhythms, compositions, melodies, raps, jingles, choral readings
Interpersonal intelligence	Good with person-to-person interactions and relationships	Group projects, group tasks, observation dialogues, conversation, debate, games, interviews
Intrapersonal intelligence	Knowledge of an inner state of being; reflective and aware	Journals, meditation, self-assessment, recording, creative expression, goal setting, affirmation, poetry
Naturalistic intelligence	Knowledge of the outside world (e.g., plants, animals, weather patterns)	Field trips, observation, nature walks, forecasting, star gazing, fishing, exploring, categorizing, collecting, identifying

Sources: Armstrong (2000a, 2000b); Gardner (1993).

• • • • • • • • • •

Sue, a student with autism, had no formal way of communicating until she was 13 years old. Before that time, she had been treated, provided therapy services, and educated as if she had a mental age of 2 years old. Mental age is often based on a person's score on an IQ test. For example, if a 14-year-old girl's score on an IQ test was the score of a "typical" or "normal" 3-year-old, she would be labeled as having the mental age of a 3-year-old. This is not a useful way to think about intelligence. When Sue acquired a form of communication called typed augmentative communication, those long-held assumptions were no longer valid. People began to realize that she was very smart. She subsequently took advanced placement classes all through her high school career, and she is now in college. (Biklen, 2005; Rubin, 2003)

• • • • • • • • • •

Because educational professionals have no real way of determining what a student understands, they should presume that every student is competent or capable. Anne Donnellan used the term *least dangerous assumption* to describe this idea: "Least dangerous assumption states that in the absence of absolute evidence, it is essential to make the assumption that, if proven to be false, would be least dangerous to the individual" (Donnellan, 1984, p. 24). In other words, it is better to presume that students are competent and that they can learn than to expect that they cannot learn.

Biklen and Burke (2006) have described this idea of presuming competence by explaining that outside observers (e.g., therapists, teachers, parents, paraprofessionals) have a choice: they can determine either that a person is competent or incompetent. The presumption of competence recognizes that no one can definitively know another person's thinking unless the other person can (accurately) reveal it. As Biklen and Burke put it, "Presuming competence refuses to limit opportunity . . . it casts the teachers, parents, and others in the role of finding ways to support the person to demonstrate his or her agency" (2006, p. 167). See Figure 5.1 for a listing of strategies for presuming competence. Also, because students without language offer unique challenges, we have included ideas about how to support those students who do not speak verbally. Please see Figure 5.2 for these ideas. This is a table that can be provided to other staff. Your role is to hand this out during professional development and make sure that every staff member who educates a student who is nonverbal receives it.

AGE-APPROPRIATE LANGUAGE

There is a tendency for people to speak down to individuals with disabilities (as if they were younger than they actually are) because of an assumption that people with disabilities are at younger developmental levels. For example, we have heard someone ask a high school student, "Do you have to use the potty?" You would not ask a high

---

- Examine your attitude—practice saying, "How can this work?" or "How can this child be successful?"
- Question your stereotypes—how someone looks, walks, or talks does not tell you about how he or she thinks and feels.
- Use age-appropriate talk—examine your tone of voice and topic.
- Support communication.
- Listen openly—work to shed judgments.
- Teach peers and others how to interpret potentially confusing behavior.
- Do not speak in front of someone as if he or she were not there.
- In conversation, refer to the person in a way that includes him or her in the conversation.
- Ask permission to share information with others.
- Be humble.
- If possible, always let the person explain for himself or herself and do not speak for him or her.
- Assume that every student will benefit from learning age-appropriate academic curriculum.
- Look for evidence of understanding.
- Support students to show understanding using their strengths.
- Design adaptations and accommodations to support access to academics.
- Be sure to acknowledge the presence of a person with a disability in the same way you would acknowledge others.
- "If you want to see competence, it helps if you look for it."

Figure 5.1. Strategies for presuming competence. (From Kasa-Hendrickson, C., & Buswell, W. [2007]. *Strategies for presuming competence.* Unpublished handout; reprinted by permission.)

"Not being able to speak is not the same thing as not having anything to say."

—*Rosemary Crossley*

A note on communication: All students who struggle with communication deserve to have a generative communication system in place so that they can express thoughts, feelings, ideas, critiques, and requests. This may include the use of sign language, an augmentative communication device, strategies to teach a person to type or point to communicate, and/or the use of eye gaze or blinking to indicate choices. While it is the right of all students to have a communication system, many students go without any way to share their thoughts.

The strategies that follow are useful in supporting a student who has an effective communication system or a student who does not have a system in place. If a student does not have a system in place, it is imperative that the team consults with a speech-language pathologist who is skilled in implementing augmentative communication systems that would meet the need of the individual child.

Keep Respect and Humanness First

- Never talk about someone as if he or she were not there. Always acknowledge the person's presence and make sure that communication in the child's presence is respectful.
- Some people may not be able to communicate that they understand what you are saying or that they are listening; assume they are listening and understand what you are talking about.
- Question your stereotypes—how someone looks, walks, or talks does not tell you about how they think and feel.
- If a student uses a wheelchair, stutters, flaps hands, or does not make eye contact, this does not mean that he or she cannot learn high-level academics, does not desire to make friends, and does not want the chance to voice independence. Work to open up opportunities.
- In conversation, refer to the person in a way that includes him or her in the conversation. For example, when Ms. Mayfield began to read the book *Splish Splash* to the class, she said, "Maya, you are going to love this book—it is all about swimming." Maya is a student who does not speak to communicate. When Ms. Mayfield shared in front of the class that Maya will enjoy this book, she taught that Maya has interests and ideas that are similar to those of her peers. In doing this, Maya did not have to respond or say anything, but her active participation and competence were made clear by her teacher's public acknowledgment.
- Ask permission to share information with others. Too often, students with disabilities do not have any privacy. Be sure not to share information on using the restroom, sexuality, health, family, embarrassing situations, and/or relationships. Ask first, and err on the side of privacy always.

Embrace a Strength-Based Attitude

- Embrace an optimistic attitude. Practice saying, "How can this work?", "How can this child be successful?"
- Work with family members to identify the student's strengths and design methods to include the student in the general education classroom using those strengths.
- Teach students to identify and use their own strengths.
- When the going gets tough, write down a list of a student's strengths and strategies to help you spring into action and begin to problem solve (see http://www.paulakluth.com/readings/inclusive-schooling/strengths-and-strategies/).

Please Act My Age: Age-Appropriate Talk and Materials

- Talk in an age-appropriate manner, using age-appropriate content. A singsong voice or a tone typically used with a young child should be reserved for babies and toddlers; be sure to check your tone of voice and the content you are talking about.
- Be sure to acknowledge the presence of a person with a disability in the same way you would acknowledge other students.

Figure 5.2. Guidelines for supporting the active participation of nonverbal students in school. (From Kasa, C., & Causton-Theoharis, J. [n.d.] *Strategies for success: Creating inclusive classrooms that work* [pp. 16–17]. Pittsburgh, PA: The PEAL Center; reprinted by permission. Retrieved from http://wsm.ezsitedesigner.com/share/scrapbook/47/472535/PEAL-S4Success_20pg_web_version.pdf)

- Let students make mistakes, get in trouble, and act out. Be sure they have the opportunity to talk and play with peers without adult interaction.

Learning to Talk to Someone Who Does Not Speak

- Be sure to acknowledge the nonverbal student's presence often. You should not go an entire lesson without saying, "Sean, I bet you'll like this part. I know you like to ski with your family," or "Megan, I see you smiling. I am sure you will like learning about volcanoes."
- Take every opportunity to teach peers how to talk to people who communicate differently. Talk about current events, age-appropriate interests, things you like to do, places to go, events around school; also, use their communication strategy to enable them to make lots of choices throughout the day: food to eat, materials to use, where to sit, what to read, what to play. Ask their opinion on various topics.

Use Communication Methods Efficiently and Often

- If a student uses a yes/no communication strategy, be sure to use this during a lesson. You can do this during a whole-group lesson by saying, "Do you all think that $5 \times 5 = 25$?" Or do this in an individual way: "Was Harry a hero in the story?" This will allow the student to use his or her yes/no strategy and be included in the lesson. If he or she answers incorrectly, then you can say, "Oh, I don't think that is quite right. Does anyone have other ideas?"
- If the student uses an augmentative communication system, you need to be sure to have them utilize it throughout the lesson. Make sure the device is ready to go with content related to the lesson so that the student can participate.

Teach Peers to Support and Understand Confusing Behavior

- Use partners during lesson activities. Model and encourage peers to talk about topics with each other. This can be done in cooperative learning groups or with peer activities such as think, pair, and share or turn and talk (see Udvari-Solner & Kluth, 2008).
- Be sure to include the student in the academic curriculum in the classroom. Assume learning is possible and ask content-related questions.
- Teach peers and others how to interpret potentially confusing behavior and support each other.

Assume Benefit from Academic Learning and Look for Understanding

- Assume that every student will benefit from learning age-appropriate academic curriculum.
- Look for evidence of understanding. This will occur in unique instances and times.
- Support students to show understanding using their strengths.
- Design adaptations and accommodations to support access to academics.

Figure 5.2.   (continued)

school student who did not have a disability that same question in that same way. Julie also has overheard someone describe a young man with Down syndrome who attends college as "a real cutie." Individuals with disabilities should be described in accordance with their actual chronological ages.

Our goal is to treat and work with students in age-appropriate ways. We once witnessed someone holding hands with a sixth-grade student in the hall. It is doubtful that it would be appropriate to hold the hand of a sixth-grade student who did not have a disability. For that very reason, it is inappropriate to hold any student's hand. This same logic holds true for having students sit on your lap, play with age-inappropriate toys, sing age-inappropriate songs, and so forth. Ask yourself how you would talk to or work with the student if she or he did not have a disability, and proceed in that manner.

PERSON-FIRST LANGUAGE

"If thoughts corrupt language, language can also corrupt thought."

—George Orwell (1946)

When describing, speaking, or writing respectfully about people who have disabilities, many people use a common language. It is called *person-first language*. The concept of person-first language is simple and is detailed in the following subsections.

The Same as Anyone Else

Think first about how you might introduce someone who does not have a disability. You might use the person's name, say how you know him or her, or describe what he or she does. The same is true for individuals with disabilities. Instead of saying, "Pat who has Down syndrome," you might say, "Pat who is in my fourth-grade class." No one should be identified by one aspect of who he or she is (especially if that aspect represents a difficulty or struggle for someone). Ask yourself why you would need to mention that the person has a disability.

Words are powerful. The ways we talk about and describe people with disabilities do not just affect our beliefs and interactions with our students; they also provide models for others who hear these descriptions.

If your own child broke his arm, would you introduce him to someone new as "my broken-armed child"? If one of the students in the school had cancer, would you expect to hear a teacher state, "She is my cancerous student"? Of course not. No one should feel ashamed about having a broken arm or having cancer, but regardless, a broken bone or malfunctioning cells do not define a person.

Avoid the Label

Would you like to be known for your medical history? Probably not. The same is true for people with disabilities. Yet, students with disabilities are invariably described with labels instead of person-first language. Have you ever heard phrases such as the *learning-disabled student, the autistic boy, that Downs child, the resource room kids,* or *the inclusion kids?*

It is important to understand the preferences of people with disabilities regarding how they would like others to speak about them. The guidelines listed in Table 5.1 come from self-advocacy groups (Disability is Natural and TASH).

COMMONLY ASKED QUESTIONS ABOUT RETHINKING STUDENTS

Q.   What if a student prefers an age-inappropriate toy or game?

A.   Often, people with disabilities have been treated as if they were younger than they are. As a result, they have been exposed to cartoons, dolls, or games to which their same-age peers have not been exposed; their peers are not likely to think these activities are cool. One option, then, is to expose the student to more age-appropriate music and activities.

Q.   Are there any exceptions to person-first language?

A.   Yes, people who are deaf often prefer the term *deaf* instead of *person with deafness*. A group called Deaf First suggests that deafness is a major component of identity, and this group prefers disability-first language. Some people with autism prefer to be called *autistic,* and some use insider language such as *autie* to describe themselves. It is inaccurate to say that all people with disabilities prefer one way over another. Person-first language serves as a helpful guideline because many advocacy groups consider it a respectful way to refer to people.

Q.   A colleague does not think the student I work with is smart. This student has a label of ID. How can I help them presume competence?

A.   This person may not perform well on standardized tests of intelligence. However, your responsibility when working with this student is to identify the student's strengths. Keep those strengths in mind. You know that every person is intelligent in different ways. You can share the student's strengths and intelligences with your colleague through stories that highlight each. This is one strategy to help your colleague presume competence.

CONCLUSION

Remember, these labels are not accurate descriptors of people. Children who have disabilities are unique individuals with unlimited potential, just like everyone else (Snow, 2008). This recognition is not only about having a good attitude or believing that all students are smart; it also will allow you to treat, support, provide services to, and work with all students in ways that promote dignity and respect. The Credo of Support poignantly reveals the importance of rethinking students (see Figure 5.3). In Chapter 6, we discuss how the ideas of dignity and respect can help facilitate social relationships.

Throughout history, people with physical and mental disabilities have been abandoned at birth, banished from society, used as court jesters, drowned and burned during The Inquisition, gassed in Nazi Germany, and still continue to be segregated, institutionalized, tortured in the name of behavior management, abused, raped, euthanized, and murdered.

Now, for the first time, people with disabilities are taking their rightful place as fully contributing citizens.

The danger is that we will respond with remediation and benevolence rather than equity and respect.

And so, we offer you

A Credo for Support

Do not see my disability as the problem.
Recognize that my disability is an attribute.

Do not see my disability as a deficit.
It is you who see me as deviant and helpless.

Do not try to fix me because I am not broken.
Support me. I can make my contribution to the community in my own way.

Do not see me as your client.
I am your fellow citizen.

See me as your neighbour.
Remember, none of us can be self-sufficient.

Do not try to modify my behavior.
Be still and listen. What you define as inappropriate may be my attempt to communicate with
　　you in the only way I can.

Do not try to change me, you have no right.
Help me learn what I want to know.

Do not hide your uncertainty behind "professional" distance.
Be a person who listens and does not take my struggle away from me by trying to make it all
　　better.

Do not use theories and strategies on me.
Be with me.
And when we struggle with each other, let that give rise to self-reflection.

Do not try to control me. I have a right to my power as a person.
What you call non-compliance or manipulation may actually be the only way I can exert some
　　control over my life.

Do not teach me to be obedient, submissive and polite.
I need to feel entitled to say No if I am to protect myself.

Figure 5.3. A credo for support. (From Kunc, N., & Van der Klift, E. [1996]. *A credo for support*. Vancouver, British Columbia: The BroadReach Centre; reprinted by permission.)

Do not be charitable towards me.
The last thing the world needs is another Jerry Lewis.
Be my ally against those who try to exploit me for their own gratification.

Do not try to be my friend. I deserve more than that.
Get to know me, we may become friends.

Do not help me, even if it does make you feel good.
Ask me if I need your help.
Let me show you how you can best assist me.

Do not admire me.
A desire to live a full life does not warrant adoration.
Respect me, for respect presumes equity.

Listen, support, and follow.

Do not work on me.
Work with me!

Figure 5.3. *(continued)*

NOTES

_____

_____

_____

_____

_____

_____

_____

_____

_____

_____

_____

_____

_____

_____

_____

_____

_____

_____

_____

_____

_____

_____

_____

_____

_____

_____

6

Providing Social Supports

Standing Back

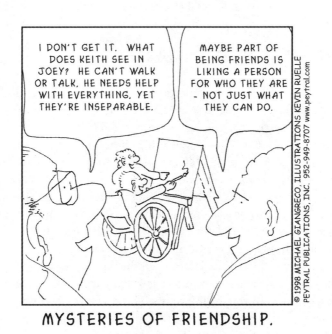

MYSTERIES OF FRIENDSHIP.

••••••••••

Seth sits down at the lunch table all by himself. Five minutes later, a few students sit at the same table. The distance between the other students and Seth makes it clear that they are not sitting with him. Seth quietly eats his lunch. Chewing carefully and using his napkin, Seth finishes his lunch and slowly packs up his belongings. He looks over at the other students. They are engaged in a conversation about their soccer team. No one says a word to Seth during lunch, and he does not talk with anyone during the entire lunch period. He puts his head down on his arm and closely examines the threads on his sweatshirt until the bell rings to indicate that lunch is over.

••••••••••

There are students like Seth at every school and in many classrooms. Often, when a student has a disability or receives support, the student's social isolation can be significant. Some students who have disabilities can undeniably have rich social lives, friendships, and social relationships. Inclusive therapy services can serve either to stigmatize and separate or to facilitate social interaction and friendship. We recognize that you already have many social strategies and this chapter is intended to provide you additional ideas to improve the social lives of students such as Seth. It will also give you ideas and suggestions for making therapy experiences social in nature. Specifically, this chapter focuses on the importance of friendships, the Velcro phenomenon, subtle and gentle supports, natural supports, your role as a bridge, supporting unstructured time, supporting structured time, teaching the rules of social interaction, and commonly asked questions.

THE IMPORTANCE OF FRIENDSHIPS

Think about your own life. How important are friendships? What do friends add to your life? For us, our own friends are critical to our quality of life. They provide entertainment; we have fun together, and they share in the joys and successes of life. Many rely on friendships—even in school. When thinking about your own schooling experience, was the motivation to get to school to see your friends? Similarly, friendships and relationships are a key part in every student's life.

"We humans want to be together. We only isolate ourselves when we are hurt by others, but alone is not our natural state" (Wheatley, 2002, p. 19). This chapter focuses on how SLPs can facilitate students' relationships with their peers and bring people together instead of hindering the students' social interactions.

Think about how it would feel if, at a certain time of day, someone came to work with you on one of your major weaknesses (e.g., balancing your checkbook). What if he or she sat down next to you during your workday and publicly worked on that skill with you, whether or not that made sense during your schedule? How would you feel? Would you feel a loss of choice? Loss of privacy? Or of freedom? What do you think your friends and co-workers would think of this new addition to your life? Do you think they would avoid you? Do you think people would flock to you? Now, imagine: how do you think your presence affects the students you support?

Sometimes, a new adult in a classroom is a magnet. Other students (particularly those in younger grades) want to connect with the adult and interact. However, the unintended consequence of side-by-side support has been widely documented—specifically, the interference with peer relationships and friendships. Giangreco, Edelman, Luiselli, and MacFarland (1997) have identified several ways in which side-by-side support (or the closeness of you to the student) can hinder students with disabilities. These include interference with the ownership (teachers see the student as "yours" when you are in the classroom, not theirs) and responsibility of general educators, separation from classmates, dependence on adults, impact on peer interactions, limitations on receiving competent instruction, loss of personal control, loss of gender identity, and interference with the instruction of other students. Other studies have determined that the close proximity of a paraprofessional or other related-service provider hinders the amount of peer interaction that occurs (Malmgren & Causton-Theoharis, 2006).

It is a careful balance. Speech-language pathology services could become a replication of the exact type of therapy that was conducted through pull-out service provision methods. This could be very embarrassing and stigmatizing to the student and is not what is meant by push-in services. The placement of one student directly next to an SLP (nearly attached) can be described as the *Velcro phenomenon*. As an SLP, it is important to avoid being "Velcroed" to a student. "Velcroing" might include sitting next to a student, pulling a student to the side for one-on-one intervention in the classroom, and so forth. There are many different alternatives to such intensive close proximity; we provide some suggestions in this chapter (see the sections Five Ways to Naturally Support Students and Six Ways to Facilitate Relationships).

THERAPY INSTEAD OF RELATIONSHIPS: WHAT IS QUALITY OF LIFE REALLY?

In an interview, Norman Kunc, a scholar who has cerebral palsy, was asked about the effect of therapy services on his life. He stated,

> Now there may be some therapists who say, "I want to help [students] function better so that they can do more things." Although that seems to be an enlightened perspective, I still have serious concerns about it because professionals mistakenly equate functioning level with quality of life and that may not be what's going on for some folks. Professionals say, "If I can help you function better, then your quality of life will improve." (Giangreco, 1996/2004, p. 37)

Michael Giangreco, who was interviewing Norman, asked, "What are your concerns with that way of thinking?" Norman responded,

> If you think about it, nondisabled people often don't equate the quality of their own lives with their ability to function in a certain way, so why apply it differently to people with disabilities? Rather than functioning level, I think most people would agree that the quality of life has to do with important personal experiences, feelings, and events, like relationships, having fun, and making contributions to the lives of other people. If you think about the most meaningful moments in life, they probably don't have to do with your functioning level. I'd bet they have

more to do with other things like getting married, the birth of your first child, your friendships, or maybe going on a spiritual retreat; they probably don't have to do with your functioning level. Ironically, developing relationships, the opportunity to make contributions to your community, even fun itself is taken away from people with disabilities in the name of trying to get them to function better to presumably improve the quality of their lives. So I didn't get to go to regular school and then I missed the opportunity to make friends. Why? Because professionals were trying to improve my quality of life by putting me in a special school where I am supposed to learn to function better. So they take away the opportunity for me to have friends and subsequently they actually interfere with the quality of my life. (Giangreco, 2004, p. 37)

This interchange should cause people to think carefully about the purpose of therapy and the human cost of therapy. It also should make educators think about ways to support students that create more opportunities for creating meaningful moments in life and rich social opportunities. At least it should cause therapists to think about how therapy services are carried out.

WHAT DOES RESEARCH SAY ABOUT VELCRO?

In a study Julie conducted with Kimber Malmgren, we observed a second-grade student named Gary as he worked in his classroom and played with his friends. Gary was supported by a paraprofessional throughout his day. During a 4-week period, Gary participated in only 32 interactions with his peers. Twenty-nine of those interactions occurred on the day when the paraprofessional was absent. Only three interactions occurred when the paraprofessional was with him, and the paraprofessional ended two of those three interactions by asking him to get back to work. Clearly, the presence of the paraprofessional had a significant impact on Gary's ability or willingness to connect with other students (Malmgren & Causton-Theoharis, 2006). Although this study was conducted with paraprofessionals, it was not the job title but the support strategies that interfered with social interactions.

HIDING IN FULL VIEW: SUBTLE, GENTLE, AND RESPECTFUL SUPPORT

At this point in the book, we move toward the "art" of providing inclusive services. Believe it or not, there is a great deal of finesse, subtlety, and elegance that goes into excellent inclusive support. This part of the job requires the most nuance, careful action, and, at times, inaction. When Jamie Burke, a college student with autism, spoke about adult support and its impact on his social interactions, he emphasized that the support he received should be subtle so that it would not interfere with his desire for a social life. He stated, "We are willing and ready to connect with other kids, and adults must quietly step into the background, camouflaging their help as a tiger who may hide in full view" (Tashie, Shapiro-Barnard, & Rossetti, 2006, p. 185). As you think about the therapy services you provide to students, find ways to camouflage your support.

FIVE WAYS TO NATURALLY SUPPORT STUDENTS

Students need to move toward independence as they grow. Providing support in natural ways is one way to help reduce dependence on support personnel. The following suggestions from Causton-Theoharis and Malmgren (2005) can help you maximize student independence and interdependence with peers and minimize student dependence on adults.

1. *Do not sit or place a chair meant for adult support next to a student.* Where you position yourself during instruction is very important. There is rarely a reason to sit directly next to a student. Even if a student needs close support because of behavior or physical support, that student probably does not need you next to him or her 100% of the time. Never have a space permanently reserved for an adult next to a student. Remove the empty chair next to the student. If you think that the expectation in a particular school or classroom is for you to sit next to a student, ask your team the following questions:

   • When is it absolutely necessary to sit next to a student to provide one-to-one support? (Examples of this type of necessary support are when providing medical assistance or lifting/transferring a student.)

   • Are there times during the day when I could provide the student with less support? If so, when?

   • When and how can we help this student increase independence?

   • When should I move away from this student?

   • Could a peer provide key supports to this student?

2. *Do not remove the student.* Friendships and relationships occur because of common experiences over long periods of time. Every time a student is removed from an inclusive classroom for therapy, that student loses potential time to interact, socialize, and learn with and from other students. If a student leaves for a sensory break, consider putting the sensory materials in the classroom; if a student is leaving because of challenging behavior, try to determine strategies that will help the student stay in the classroom (for strategies for working with students who have challenging behavior, see Chapter 8).

3. *Encourage peer support.* If a student asks for your help with something, have the student ask a peer instead. Make this the norm for all students. One useful way to set this up is to have all students follow the rule "Ask three before me." Set up partnerships during instructional time. Have students work together. Set up play partners, transition partners (partners for walking to and from classes), choice time partners, lunchtime partners, math partners, and so forth. Make sure the student you are supporting has a choice about

who he or she selects as a partner. Giving students the skills to seek peer support promotes a valid and important lifelong skill.

4. *Encourage independence and interdependence.* If a student is able to complete a task in your presence without adult support, have him or her complete the task without supervision the next time. For example, Chloe is working on verbally responding in the large classroom setting when called on. She is able to complete the task with a prompt from the SLP of "go ahead and share." The next day, the team has a written sticky note that says "go ahead and share." This time the general education teacher asks a question and then points to the sticky note as a cue. When Chloe is successful with the sticky note, next a peer is told she can help to cue her by pointing to the note. Last, Chloe is independent with the skill, but she is next taught to "phone a friend" or ask for help if she is called on and does not know the answer.

Continually ask yourself what the next step is that will enable a student to become more independent and less dependent on adult support. If a student will still need assistance, consider having interdependence (or successfully completing the task with other students) be the goal. By the end of the year, sometimes Chloe would ask her table mates for help if she was called on, but at least she did not require adult support and instead had a way to ask for help and initiate communication with peers.

5. *Fade your cues.* One of the simplest yet most effective ways to increase interaction for students is to fade assistance. Fading assistance means actually reducing the type and level of support given to a student in a systematic way. Reducing support promotes independence, interdependence, and interaction with peers. Take a look at the cuing structure list shown in Table 6.1. The goal with this structure is always to move away from the most obtrusive supports (those on top) to the least obtrusive supports (those on the bottom) for students whenever possible (Doyle, 2008).

Providing natural or unobtrusive supports is a very important first step toward helping students feel like everyone else. The next step in helping students connect with one another is to facilitate relationships and assist students with positive social interactions by becoming a bridge linking students and their peers.

YOUR ROLE AS A BRIDGE BETWEEN STUDENTS WITH DISABILITIES AND THEIR PEERS

You can become a bridge connecting students; you can blend in, provide more natural supports, and facilitate relationships among students. The following subsection offers six ways to help students relate to one another to form lasting friendships.

Table 6.1. Types of support

Type of support (listed from most intrusive to least)	Definition	Example
Full physical	Direct and physical assistance used to support a student	Hand-over-hand assistance while a student writes his or her name
Partial physical	Physical assistance provided for some of the total movement required for the activity	Putting a zipper into the bottom portion and beginning to pull up; the student then pulls the zipper up the rest of the way
Modeling	A demonstration of what the student is to do	The adult does an art project; the student uses the art project as a model.
Direct verbal	Verbal information provided directly to the student	"Josh, stand up now."
Indirect verbal	A verbal reminder that prompts the student to attend to or think about what is expected	"Josh, what should happen next?"
Gestural	A physical movement to communicate or accentuate a cue (e.g., head nod, thumbs up, pointing)	Adult points to the agenda written on the board.
Natural	Providing no cue; allowing the ordinary cues that exist in the environment to help the student know what to do	The bell rings for class. The teacher asks students to move to the rug. A message on the chalkboard reads, "Turn to page 74."

Source: Doyle (2008).

Six Ways to Facilitate Relationships

These ideas have been modified from Causton-Theoharis and Malmgren (2005):

1. *Highlight similarities among students.* In a general education classroom, students are continually talking and sharing stories about things not related to the curriculum (e.g., hobbies, extracurricular activities). Become conscious of conversations going on around the student and point out similarities. For example, as students are talking about T-ball, you might say, "Oh, Josh's sister plays T-ball." Or, as students are settling down with their library books, you might point out similarities among their books: "The two of you both selected books about computers. You can sit together and compare your books."

2. *Help students invite each other to socialize.* Some students are very eager to socialize but do not know how to approach other students. It can be helpful for an SLP to be proactive about all of the potential social situations that occur throughout the school day. Think ahead about social possibilities, and ask the student, "Who do you want to play with at recess today?" "How can you ask them?" "Who do you want to sit next to in study hall?" If you have a student who is nonverbal, provide a picture list of the students in the class and help the student program his or her device to ask a friend. An index card that says, "Do you want to play with me?" or "Will you be my partner?" can be very useful in such situations.

3. *Provide behavioral supports that are social in nature.* When a student is rewarded for doing a good job, make the reception of the reward something social. This way, the reward can be more fun for all involved, and it will have the added benefit of allowing students to learn and practice social interaction. Some examples of these types of interactive behavioral supports follow:

- Shoot baskets with a friend.

- Eat lunch with a friend.

- Make bead necklaces with a friend during study hall.

- Play a computer game with a friend.

- Go to the library and read with a friend.

- Make an art project before school with a friend.

4. *Provide responsibilities that are interactive and collaborative.* Students are commonly assigned responsibilities within the classroom and school environments. This is done to help students contribute to the classroom community and to build a sense of belonging. SLPs can be key participants in helping create partners for these tasks and embedding speech and language goals into the jobs. For example, change the job chart in the classroom so that all jobs are done with buddies. When jobs arise in the classroom, ask students to do the jobs together: "Sue and Joryann, can you please pass out these papers?" Much more spontaneous communication will occur when students are expected to work together.

5. *Help other students understand.* Peers are much more likely to interact with students if they understand necessary information about each other. Provide honest answers to students' questions. Chelsea once heard a little girl ask, in reference to another student's FM audio device, "Why does he wear that thing on his head?" The educator said that it was private and that she should get back to work. The student got back to work, but an important question had been left unanswered. In the mind of the little girl, the subject was not to be talked about. As an unintended result, the student using the FM system might seem taboo. Your job is not to share confidential information about students with their peers. However, there are times when providing basic information about a student or the type of support they are receiving may be helpful to the student. If you are unsure about whether to share information, ask the student and the special education service coordinator. As a more proactive way of addressing such subjects, some teaching teams have decided to bring their classes together to talk about what makes everyone special. For example, the students in one middle school classroom all listed things that made them unique. Then, they posted this information on a bulletin board. Some students included "I live with my grandmother" or "I speak two languages." One student in this class wrote, "I know sign language." This type of conversation can be used to describe specific behaviors or the accommodations that a student receives. Information can be shared about

how and when to assist a particular student (e.g., do not talk in a baby voice, do ask whether he needs help). Before initiating a discussion of this type, make sure the student is comfortable with the plan, and involve all parties in deciding what information the student wants to share.

6. *Get out of the way!* When a conversation among students has begun, give the students space so that a natural conversation can occur; eventually, a relationship may evolve. Think about where you should stand; try to be as unobtrusive to the student as possible. If you remain close, it will be clear to everyone around that you are there, creating an invisible barrier between other students and the one you are supporting. Instead, while fading, move away and focus your attention on something else.

SUPPORTING UNSTRUCTURED TIME

Social interaction occurs at all times during the school day. Unstructured times are some of the most important times to provide support that will help students connect to one another. Examples of key times are listed in the following subsections, with some suggestions that should be useful.

Before and After School

Students spend a lot of time traveling to and from school. This is a perfect time to facilitate social interaction. For before and after school, help the family find a travel partner or someone in the neighborhood to walk to school or ride the bus with the student. Many SLPs find the before or after school time perfect for supporting skills like social communication and swallowing during breakfast at school.

In the Hallway

Have walking partners in the hallway between classes. A team that Chelsea worked with had the students engage in partner Simon Says. During this 5-minute transition, the SLP had students doing mirror activities with their partners as they walked down the hall. For example, she had them stick out tongue, say tongue twisters, repeat silly sounds, and more. Many of these were skills that she had once practiced in her therapy room and now everyone was benefiting from extra practice and transitions were more fun. Not only was this a creative way to infuse speech-language therapy skills, but all of the students loved and requested this transition game. Another team had a student push a student named Samantha in her wheelchair while another student walked alongside her. This allowed Samantha to have some space from an adult and a chance to converse. If a student does not use speech, program the device that the student uses to have common chatty phrases such as "How's it going?" As the student moves through the hallway, he or she can start or initiate interactions.

At Lunchtime

Many SLPs work with students during lunch. Be thoughtful about how direct services at lunchtime affect natural interactions. Whenever possible, avoid direct side-by-side services during lunch. Where students sit at lunch is very important. Do not have students with disabilities sit together at one table. Instead, help students to select lunch places at which they will feel the most comfortable and, at the same time, have increased likelihood of interacting with peers. Some schools create interest tables at which students' interests are printed on table tent cards (e.g., chess, Pokémon, rainforest animals). Students sit at tables that interest them and can freely converse about their preferred topic. Other schools have "lunch bunches." Organizing a lunch bunch is a useful way to help a student who struggles with social interaction during the lunch period and perfect for providing some types of services. A lunch bunch involves gathering a group of students during the lunch period for a particular purpose (e.g., planning the end-of-year picnic, creating a class yearbook). This mixed group of students (not all students with disabilities) can meet weekly to complete the task. At the end of the year, the lunch bunch might celebrate the accomplishments with a pizza party. The objective is to bring students together in a more intimate setting, to foster social interaction and help form friendships.

Music can be provided at lunchtime to create a calming atmosphere. A team in one school employed this strategy because Jonah, the student with autism whom they supported, had found the lunchroom to be overloading to his senses. After asking him what kind of music he would like to have on, the team piped Beatles music into the lunchroom, providing a calming atmosphere for all students. Best of all, Jonah was able to stay in the lunchroom and connect with other students.

At Free or Choice Time

Help students choose the activities they want to do and which peers they want to participate with them. In third grade, the ability to initiate conversation to join a group during recess is crucial. The SLP had a 5-minute conference with Josh to brainstorm three ways to join a group to play with during recess. The SLP took the ideas from this conversation and wrote a social script that Josh placed in his locker. While getting his lunch and coat each day, he reviewed the social script to prepare for recess. The SLP supported Josh to have ideas to initiate interaction with his peers.

To Select Partners

The words students least like to hear in classrooms are "Find a partner." Inevitably, as students clamor to work with their friends, someone will be left out and need a partner. If that happens, do not become the student's partner. Instead, help the student find a friend. It can be far more helpful to determine partners ahead of time. One very thoughtful team, tired of seeing the same scenario occur with Kristin repeatedly during math class, came up with a new solution. They used purposeful partnering to ensure that each student, including Kristin, had 12 different partners, one for each hour. This solution created partners who would remain constant so that students did not have to feel left out. Using a Clock Buddies sheet found online (Jones, 1998–2006; see Figure 6.1), they purposefully set up partners for the rest of the year by having students sign up on the Clock Buddies sheet. From that point on, when the teacher would say, "Find your 2:00 partner," Kristin knew exactly who her partner would be, and she was able to participate successfully in the math center.

SUPPORT DURING INSTRUCTIONAL TIME

During instructional time, walk around the room, supporting all students and answering everyone's questions. It can be very stigmatizing to be the only one receiving help.

CLOCK BUDDIES

Figure 6.1. A Clock Buddies sign-up sheet. (From Jones, R.C. [1998–2006]. *Strategies for reading comprehension: Clock buddies.* Retrieved from http://www.readingquest.org/strat/clock_buddies.html; reprinted by permission.)

The best scenario is one in which you provide support to the entire class, with none of the students thinking that you are there to help a specific student. Avoid calling yourself "Claire's therapist." Instead, refer to yourself as someone who supports everyone. As soon as a student has gotten started, do not hover. Give the student space to work and make mistakes, just like everyone else. Have the student request help in the same way that everyone else does. If you must redirect a student, do so quietly. Also praise quietly. Each of these aspects is important, and your support should be as unobtrusive and gentle as possible.

To ensure that all students come into contact with a student with disabilities, you can move instructional materials to the student instead of asking the other students to go to a certain station or object. Julie witnessed a team do this beautifully with Alex, a student in kindergarten who used a wheelchair. All of the students were moving over to a globe to gather information. The team decided to move the globe over to Alex's desk, and, as the students came over to look at it, many of them interacted with Alex.

TEACH KIDS THE RULES OF SOCIAL INTERACTION

Many children or students struggle with how to interact with others. They think they are playing a game for which they do not know the rules. If you are working with a child who feels this way, teach him or her the rules explicitly. However, do not teach the rules in isolation or in a separate room with only students who have disabilities. Instead, use everyday moments in the classroom and on the playground to artfully teach students how to interact with one another. There are many resources available to help you. Carol Gray has written several books on writing social stories for students with autism and on drawing social situations in cartoon form to help students understand social rules (see Gray, 2013). For other ideas, ask your team of teachers or do some research online. Educators should not assume loneliness is part of the schooling experience; they can intervene and help students make and maintain friendships.

COMMONLY ASKED QUESTIONS ABOUT SOCIAL SUPPORTS

Q. This student's challenging behavior makes other kids not want to be around him or her. What could I do about that?

A. First, assume that the student is worthy of friendships and relationships. Help support the student in a way that will both minimize the behavior and help others understand the behavior. One student, Kenny, used to rock back and forth when he felt anxious, and this behavior looked strange to Kenny's peers. Simply explaining to the other students what the behavior meant allowed one bright student to ask Kenny, "What can I do to help you stop rocking?" Kenny typed out a response with his SLP: "Let me put my hand on your shoulder." From that moment on, Kenny's peers helped him to manage his rocking behavior by asking, "Do you want to lean on me?"

Q. I understand why I should fade my support, but I worry that will not count as student contact minutes. What can I do while I am fading my support?

A. This is a common concern. Direct contact minutes does not mean you are in direct contact with students (e.g., touching the student, hand-over-hand support, sitting at their table). Instead it means they are engaged in learning experiences that you have helped to construct with your expertise. When they are practicing a skill (e.g., verbal turn taking), you can get students started and walk around the room helping others. When you return, you can help cue the students and continue moving. When moving away from a student, you can support other students, prepare for an upcoming class by creating modifications, or take data.

CONCLUSION

Seth was introduced at the beginning of this chapter. Seth is a student who struggles with social interactions. The biggest detriment to his social life is that he has an adult supporting him all school day long and he is pulled out continually for therapies. Friendships and relationships are critical to Seth's development and quality of life. This is true for all students, and for those who receive therapy, care needs to be taken to ensure maximum inclusion and opportunities for social interaction. SLPs are uniquely positioned to support students inclusively, because so much of the work relates to human communication. The suggestions mentioned in this chapter are meant to support your efforts to include students in the social aspects of school. The next chapter focuses on providing services during academic instructional time. However, be mindful that in the inclusive classroom you often will need to provide both social and academic supports at the same time.

NOTES

7

Providing Academic Supports

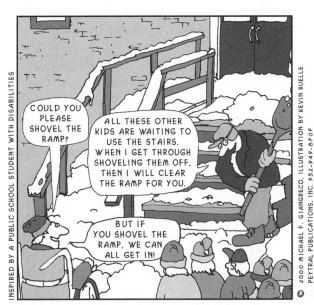

CLEARING A PATH
FOR PEOPLE WITH SPECIAL NEEDS
CLEARS THE PATH FOR EVERYONE!

"My goal is to provide modeling with the language and also the fluency piece when providing classroom-based services. It helps everyone—the teacher and the paraprofessional—to see how I am prompting Josie to improve her language and fluency. Then, it's also during the planning that I am making key contributing decisions, along with the teacher and special education teacher, about Josie's day to make sure she's practicing these skills throughout the day."

—Pat (SLP)

We both use several modifications throughout the day to be successful. For example, Julie sets her alarm to wake up. She goes on a brisk walk before the demands of the day begin; this improves her ability to sit for long periods of time at work. Chelsea wakes up early to allow herself an hour of uninterrupted time to write before anyone else in the house wakes up, before the phone rings, and before checking e-mail. Both Chelsea and Julie use an electronic calendar to keep daily appointments. Chelsea has a binder with colorful sections she uses as a daily to-do list. There is a section for each of the big projects she is working on. She crosses each item off as she completes it. Julie typically writes her daily to-do list in a notebook. She prioritizes each item by writing numbers in the left-hand margin of the list. We both use systems to help us to organize our lives in efficient ways. When Julie cleans her house, she sets an alarm for 15 minutes and races around the house to see how much she can get done before setting the alarm again for the next room. Our point is this: All individuals need their environments, time schedules, and behavior modified or adapted to allow them to be successful members of society.

SLPs who work in school settings have the goal to provide the needed speech sound production, resonance, voice, fluency, language, cognition, feeding, and swallowing supports that allow children to be successful in academics. This chapter does just that; that is, we discuss accommodations, modifications, and adaptations that enable students with disabilities to benefit from general education. We describe general, content-specific, and environmental strategies and discuss the topic of assistive technology.

As an SLP, your expertise is intended to support students to participate in and benefit from special education and participate in educational activities related to communication, language, fluency, voice, and swallowing. You provide modifications, adaptations, and skill development that allow students to succeed in communication efforts throughout the school environment. Speech-language services in schools are provided within the context of the child's educational program. As such, speech-language service provision happens authentically within the school environment where the need occurs. This can be a formidable task.

According to Part B of IDEA 2004 (PL 108-446), speech-language pathology is a "related service" for children ages 3–21 who require support to benefit from special education and "who have diagnosed disabilities that are physical, behavior/psychosocial, cognitive, or other delay that interfere with the child's ability to benefit from special education" (§602[26][A]). IDEA 2004 recognizes that education for students with disabilities is effective when it is based on high expectations, participation, and progress in the general education curriculum alongside peers without disabilities to the maximum extent possible. Under IDEA 2004, special education means "specially designed instruction . . . to meet the unique needs of a child with a disability" (34 C.F.R. §300.39). This specially designed instruction "means adapting, as appropriate to the needs of an eligible child . . . the content, methodology, or delivery of instruction" in order 1) "to address the unique needs of the child that result from the child's disability" and 2) "to ensure access of the child to the general curriculum, so that the child can meet the educational standards within the jurisdiction of the public agency that apply to all children" (IDEA 2004; 34 C.F.R. §300.39[b][3]). SLPs have expertise about specific student needs that is immensely beneficial to the educational team in ensuring a student has purposeful access to the general education curriculum and "specially designed" special education.

This chapter will familiarize you with several modifications and specific ways to adapt learning experiences to meet the speech-language therapy and academic needs of the students on your caseload. This chapter first describes general strategies that will enable you to support students, then discusses content-specific ideas and environmental strategies, and, finally, suggests strategies that can help you work across all content areas. Consider reading this chapter with your entire educational team.

Figure 7.1 shows a general cycle of support, which has been adapted from one developed by Mary Beth Doyle (2008).

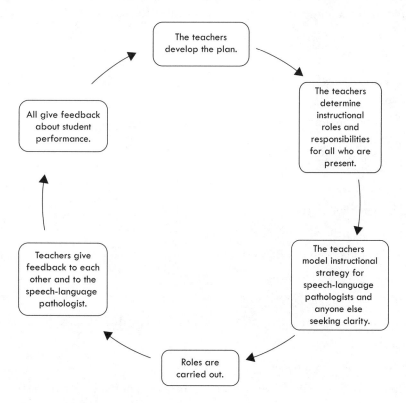

Figure 7.1. General cycle of support. (From Doyle, M.B. [2008]. *The paraprofessional's guide to the inclusive classroom: Working as a team* [3rd ed., p. 58]. Baltimore, MD: Paul H. Brookes Publishing Co.; adapted by permission.)

ACCOMMODATIONS, MODIFICATIONS, AND ADAPTATIONS

The following information about the differences between modifications and adaptations comes from the PEAK Parent Center (n.d.) in Colorado Springs, Colorado. *Accommodations* and *modifications* are adaptations made to the environment, curriculum, instruction, or assessment practices that enable students with disabilities to be successful learners and to participate actively with other students in the general education classroom and in schoolwide activities.

Accommodations are changes in how a student gains access to information and demonstrates learning. Accommodations do not substantially change the instructional level, content, or performance criteria. The changes are made to provide a student with equal access to learning and equal opportunity to show what he or she knows and can do. Accommodations can include changes in presentation, response format and procedures, instructional strategies, time and scheduling, environment, equipment, and architecture.

Modifications are changes in what a student is expected to learn. The changes are made to provide a student with opportunities to participate meaningfully and productively along with other students in classroom and school learning experiences. Modifications include changes in instructional level, content, and performance criteria. Figure 7.2 provides a list of the top 10 worst classroom modifications.

The following lists contain examples of accommodations and modifications that can be provided in general education classrooms. IEP teams determine accommodations and modifications that meet the unique and individual needs of their students.

Accommodations

- Recording device for presentations, allowing for self-monitoring of phonation and pitch
- PVC fluency phones during independent and buddy reading
- Use of calming strategies, mediated breathing prior to speech production
- Test taken orally
- Large-print textbooks
- Additional time to take test
- A locker with an adapted lock
- Weekly home–school communication tool, such as a notebook or daily log book
- Peer support for notetaking
- Lab sheets with highlighted instructions
- Graph paper to assist in organizing and lining up math problems
- Tape-recorded lectures
- Use of a computer for writing
- Whiteboard (see Table 7.1 for a list of 16 uses for a portable whiteboard)
- Use of a variety of tablet computer applications (see Table 7.2 for a list of possible speech-language apps)

Table 7.1. Sixteen ideas for using a portable whiteboard to support communication[a]

Use	Description
If–then board	Write a phrase such as, "If you finish your math, then you may choose a friend for computer buddies."
Sentence starters	Examples: Wilber probably felt . . . This weekend I . . . If the moon were made of . . .
To-do lists	Example: 1. Silent reading 2. Two questions 3. Partner reading 4. Snack time
Reminders	Example: Please keep your voice at a level 2.
Cartoon conversations	Drawn conversations[b]
Visual notes or mental movie	Students can draw the big ideas from the lecture or the read-aloud.
Written directions for things only presented orally	Examples: Turn to page 321. What kind of matter is toothpaste?
Response board	Have the student write the answer and hold up the whiteboard.
Parking lot	A place for student to write ideas while waiting to share verbally
Drawing space	A place for a student to draw during downtime or discussion time
Graphic organizers	Draw a Venn diagram or other graphic organizer to allow the student to organize thoughts for a writing project or conversation.
Quick-pick boards	ABCD or Yes/No or T/F can be written and the student can point.
Writing model	Begin the student's sentence as a model to help him or her get started.
Visual model of voice pitch	Demonstrate voice pitch with a line. For a monotone voice use a straight line, and for questions use a curved line that gradually goes up.
Visual models of the spatial concepts	Draw a picture for in, above, over, and so forth.
Written conversation with a peer	Example: A peer writes, "How was your weekend?" and the student responds in pictures or words.

[a]A small wipe-off whiteboard can be an excellent tool when supporting a student in the general education classroom. It is versatile and can be used to support activities in real time.
[b]See Carol Gray's (2013) cartoon conversations for activity guidelines.

Modifications

- Highlighted step-by-step written directions (as opposed to oral directions)
- Picture cues that go with verbal communication for daily choices
- An outline in place of an essay for a major project
- Picture communication symbol choices on tests
- Written lines combined with visual scripts for Readers Theater
- Alternative books or materials on the same theme or topic
- Spelling support from a computerized spell-check program
- Word bank of choices for answers to test questions
- Use of a calculator on a math test
- Film or video supplements in place of text
- Questions reworded using simplified language
- Projects substituted for written reports
- Important words and phrases highlighted

Table 7.2. Thirteen must-have applications to support communication

Application (app)	Description
StoryPals	This app fosters story comprehension. Features include text-to-speech and word highlighting to aid in comprehension.
Puppet Pals	Students select their own characters for digital puppets and a background. Work on social cues of language, conversations, and comprehension with this app.
ArtikPix	This app focuses on speech articulation. Features include group scoring for cooperative groups.
Time Timer	This app turns the passage of time as an abstract concept into a visual reminder that students can actually see.
iBrainstorm	iBrainstorm is the perfect app for idea generation and figuring out possible solutions. Record ideas on colored Post-it notes that can be organized into hierarchies.
Toontastic	This is a great storytelling app that bolsters students' language skills. Create a graphic organizer, draw the setting and character traits, animate the screen, audio record voices for the characters, and publish the story online.
Proloquo2Go	This app offers an augmentative and alternative communication option for students who are nonverbal or have difficulty speaking. Features include text-to-speech function.
Articulate it!	This app includes phonemes and over 1,200 photo cards that allow the speech-language pathologist to target specific phonemes, phonological processing, or articulation skills.
ConversationBuilder	This app allows students to practice multiple exchanges in conversation settings that will allow students to have better interactions with peers.
iCommunicate	Use this to design visual schedules and choices boards that are individualized for students.
Caseload Tracker	Stay organized with this app that allows you to keep track of individualized education programs, meetings, evaluation, and eligibility due dates.
Pocket SLP	These customizable cards have 2,100 target phonemes and illustrative examples of how to produce sounds.
Bla Bla Bla	This app shows students how to moderate their voice volume and provides good visual feedback of voice level.

Note: Tablet computer apps provide engaging strategies to support students' speech sound production, voice, fluency, and language during the natural school context. All of these apps should be used to augment and support the general education content within the general education setting. A caution here is not to use these apps in a pull-out fashion. Remember that the purpose of special education and related services is to gain access to the general education content.

Deciding which accommodations and/or modifications to use is a process that depends on the assignment and needs of each individual student. This process will be determined by the educational team, and you have a wealth of expertise to bring to these decisions. As an SLP, you are expected to have a role in designing the accommodations and/or modifications throughout a student's school experience. However, you may not necessarily be the primary person who implements each. When you provide direct services within the classroom, you will have a primary role in the implementation process. At other times, you may support the educational team in the design process during a weekly meeting. Through indirect consultant services, your expertise regarding speech and language needs will be utilized. When the appropriate adaptations are made, all students can have meaningful access to the general education curriculum (PEAK Parent Center, n.d.).

10. The seventh grade class is doing math, but one student is using *Sesame Street* blocks to work on counting.

9. The class is watching a video, but one student who is blind is sent out of the room because she cannot see.

8. The classroom is arranged with desks in groups of five, but one student is seated in a group with only two desks, one for him and one for his assistant.

7. While the rest of the high school class is doing reports on nutrition, one student is given a tub of dry beans and rice to "explore."

6. Fourth-grade students are adding adjectives to sentences, but because the speech-language pathologist has not yet put adjectives on one student's communication board, the student does not participate in this lesson.

5. During silent reading, the speech-language pathologist takes one student to the back of the classroom to work on articulation.

4. Because one student has dressing goals on her individualized education program, she puts on and takes off her shoes two times when she gets ready for gym class.

3. Because one student does not yet read, she listens to a music tape while the teacher reads aloud to the class.

2. A student who types to communicate is provided with a device *only* during language arts class.

1. A 12-year-old student goes with the second-grade class to physical education because his gross motor skills are "at that level."

Figure 7.2. Top 10 worst classroom modifications.

GENERAL STRATEGIES

"Working with the team to make sure Zach has the needed communication and language supports and accommodations across his day to allow him to succeed is really what my job is all about."

—Jane (SLP)

Some strategies for providing academic support include focusing on strengths, asking the student, keeping expectations high, breaking tasks into smaller steps, and providing extended time.

Focus on Strengths

When providing support to students, it is easy for educators to become overwhelmed by what a student cannot do. For example, when providing support to Steven, a third grader with Down syndrome, it was easy to think, "Steven does not read and does not talk; how am I to help him understand the science content in this chapter?" It helps to reframe your thinking and ask yourself what the student *can* do. Focus instead on the student's strengths; with Steven, you might think, "Steven is a very social guy. He can easily comprehend big ideas. He is masterful at drawing what he knows and labeling parts. He also can answer questions."

We focused on Steven's strengths of listening, social interaction, and understanding main ideas. When other students were required to quietly read the chapter from the science book, Steven's partner read the chapter aloud. At the end of each section in the text, Steven and his partner were required to say something about the section, and Steven, as he listened, worked on a drawing depicting the big ideas from that section. Steven and his partner then asked each other questions about the section and the drawing. This worked so well for Steven and his partner that the teacher decided to have the entire class read the science text that way for the rest of the year.

Ask the Student

After discussing the student's support requirements with the general education and special education teachers, you should consult the student. One strategy is to openly ask the student what type of language and communication works well. Seeing the student as the expert in his or her own needs is crucial. Tailor your speech, language, and communication support around the student's recommendations.

Keep Expectations High

If a student has a disability, it does not mean that the student cannot complete assignments and projects in the same way as anyone else. Before attempting to modify or alter a student's assignment, ask yourself whether the assignment actually needs any changes. Too often, educational professionals overmodify for students or decide to make the same modification for every student with the same disability. Sometimes, the best thing to do for a student is not to change your expectations for him or her but, instead, to change the type or level of support.

Break Tasks into Smaller Steps

For some students, it might be useful to break tasks into smaller parts. For example, one student preferred having a to-do list posted on her desk for any independent work time. The team would write down the big tasks that needed to be completed, and the student would complete them independently and cross out each task. If you have a student who does not read, you could draw a picture list and have the student cross out each picture as he or she completes each task.

Extend Time on Tasks

Many students can complete the same work as anyone else if they have extra time. In these cases, it may be helpful to slowly decrease the time allotted for certain tasks. Or, if the other students have an hour to complete a test, allow the student to take the test in parts—one part on the first day, the second part on the next.

Present a Limited Amount of Information on a Page

Some students prefer to see less information at once. The layout of information should be clean and free of distraction. Adequate white space, for example, can make an assignment appear less confusing. This modification can easily be made by copying different segments of an assignment onto different pages. In addition, Wite-Out tape helps limit certain distracting information or pictures. Then, when the item is photocopied, the student has less information to wade through. An index card or a word window (i.e., a piece of cardboard with a small rectangular window covered with cellophane that allows students to see one line of text or one word at a time) can also help students eliminate information as they read by themselves.

Offer Support, Do Not Just Give It

Do not assume that a student needs help. If a student is struggling, encourage him or her to ask a peer first. If the student is still struggling, ask, "Can I help you get started?" If the student says, "No," respect his or her wishes.

Use a Soft Voice

Receiving support is not always a comfortable thing. It also can be distracting to classmates. Therefore, when students are working, use a soft voice.

Make Things Concrete

Many students need concrete examples, such as pictures or videos that support the concepts taught in class. Having someone on the team search the school library and Internet for pictures and videos to support learning is helpful. The teacher can then incorporate these teaching aids into mini-lectures and teaching centers. Use of visual supports benefits not only the students with disabilities, but everyone in the class.

Teach Organizational Skills to Everyone

It is common for students with and without disabilities to struggle with organization. In a seventh-grade classroom, performing binder checks at the end of each class to make sure the notes are in the correct color-coded spot as students leave the room is helpful. In one example we witnessed, this supported not only Adam, who chronically struggled with keeping things organized, but countless others who needed similar support. Another team we know of made a checklist of all the items students needed to take home each day. These lists were made available for any student to use.

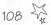

Change the Materials

Sometimes, all a student needs for success is a different type of material. A change in writing utensil or size or type of paper can make a substantial difference for a student. For example, every time Brett was expected to write, he would put his head down on the desk or angrily break pencils. The team of teachers, therapists, and paraprofessionals who supported the classroom met and discussed the potential reasons for Brett's behavior and how the team might make writing more pleasant for him. As a result of this conversation, the SLP recommended letting all students have an optional two-minute conference to brainstorm their writing plan with a partner. When this choice was provided, Brett chose to conference with a friend, telling him the details of his story. This allowed him the executive functioning support needed and, when he sat down, he immediately wrote two paragraphs. He later explained that he would get nervous if he saw "a whole blank piece of paper" and that "writing conferences help sort my brain and give me something to write about."

Use a Timer

Timers can be useful for students who like to know how long tasks will take or who need help organizing their time. For some students, visual timers, or timers in which the student can see how much time is left, can be particularly useful. For Izzy, the timer helps him know when the transition is occurring and also gives him an important responsibility.

··········

Izzy is a kindergarten student. Whenever transitions in the classroom occur, he has loud tantrums. Because of Izzy's difficulty with transitions, his therapist recommends to use a timer to alert him when the transitions are coming. Izzy's teacher hands him an old track timer and tells him that he is in charge of letting the other students know when it is cleanup time. After first practicing with the timer, Izzy takes his responsibility very seriously. He walks around from group to group, reminding the kindergartners that there are only "5 minutes until cleanup time . . . 4 minutes . . . 3. . . ." He continues to remind his friends until the timer goes off. He then shouts, "Clean up everyone!"

··········

Preteach

Preteaching big ideas such as vocabulary or major concepts can be useful for many students. Preteaching should be done before a concept is "officially" taught to the rest of the class. You may introduce a concept, term, or idea to a student before the rest of the students learn it. For example, as the students were preparing for a magnet lab, Erik taught some of the key science vocabulary to Brett before the lesson. Brett entered the magnet lab understanding the terms *attract* and *repel*. This allowed Brett to come into the class prepared and more confident.

Peer Support

Peer support is one of the best ways to support students. Have all the students work in teams or partnerships. Tell students that their job is to help each other. However, some caution is necessary regarding peer support. Do not set up "helping relationships"—for example, Sonja always helps Jose. Instead, encourage students to help each other. Figure out times when Jose can help Sonja and others in the classroom.

Use Movement

Most students need to move their bodies often. When asking students to memorize discrete concepts or pieces of information, use visual cues, signs, or movements. Many students who have trouble memorizing can be helped by using movements or visual cues. Challenge students to come up with their own movements that match the concepts of specific words. For example, one sixth-grade teacher had her class do "spelling aerobics." When spelling words, if the letters were "tall letters" (e.g., *t, l, b*), the students would stand up tall and put their arms up; if letters were "short" (e.g., *o, e, a*), the students would put their hands on their hips; and, if letters hung below the line (e.g., *p, g, q*), the students would touch their toes. For instance, to spell the word *stop,* the students would touch their waists, reach up, touch their waists, and then touch their toes. What makes this particular example so powerful is that the movement is purposeful and connected to the content.

Content-Specific Strategies

Tables 7.3 and 7.4 detail modifications and adaptations for different types of content and activities that are commonly used across content areas.

Remember, you will be responsible for recommending ideas and consulting with the teacher. You should know these types of modifications and how best to use them with students who need speech and language services and supports. If you see an idea in Table 7.3 that you would like to try with a student, talk to the team to decide whether it would be an effective strategy. Discuss how to use it, when to use it, and when you might fade the strategy or idea.

Commonly Occurring Activities Across Content Areas

Support can look very different for students in different content areas. Sometimes, a different teacher is responsible for each content area, and this can result in different expectations. Some students prefer certain subjects and perform better in them. For example, Ricky enjoyed music, so he needed almost no support in that class. He would enter the music room, gather his folder and instrument, and be ready to go. In science, he did not seem fond of the teacher or the subject, and he therefore needed more support to get started with tasks. Although a student's support might look different from class to class, teachers use similar activities across different subject areas. Table 7.4 highlights activities that are used commonly across subjects. Teachers may require students to do any number of these things throughout the day. Nonetheless,

Table 7.3.   Content-specific modifications

In this subject	Consider these modifications, adaptations, and accommodations
Reading/language arts	Listen to digital books. Read with a peer. Follow along with a word window. Read from a computer with headphones. Work with a peer and have him or her summarize. Read enlarged print. Use CCTV (closed circuit TV)—a video magnifier that enlarges the font. Rewrite stories in more simple language. Use books with repetitive texts.
Mathematics	Calculators Touch math (each number has the correct number of dots on the actual number) Hundreds charts Number lines Flash cards Count stickers Manipulatives (e.g., Unifix cubes, counting chips) Worksheet modified with easier-to-read numbers Pictures or visuals Larger cubes Chart paper to keep track of columns Talking calculator Numbered dice instead of dotted dice Real-world problems—problems with students' names in them
Physical education	Different-sized sporting equipment Silent activities (for those who are sensitive to noise) Choice stations Change the size of the court
Art	Choice of materials Bigger/smaller materials Slant board Precut materials Stencils Smocks and aprons with pockets Gloves for kids who do not like to get messy Wiki sticks Posted steps about the process Modified scissors
Science	Hands-on experiences Teacher demonstration A role play Guest speaker Posted steps indicating the process
Social studies	Highlighters or highlighting tape A way to connect the content to self DVDs Visuals Maps A written task card (a card with a step-by-step process on it)
Music	Songs in the student's native language Instruments Signs while singing Rhythms to clap out Tapes/CDs of music to practice at home Music videos to watch

Table 7.4. Common activities and supports

When the students are asked to	Consider providing students
Sit and listen	Visuals to look at Movement breaks An FM system (that amplifies the teacher's voice) A rug or mat to help determine where to be An object to signify who is speaking (e.g., a talking stick) A ball to sit on Choice about where to sit A focus object for students to hold or manipulate A signal to start listening The book that is being read A topic bag—filled with objects that relate to the content A job to do (help another student, write ideas on the board)
Present orally	Choice about the supports necessary Note cards Visuals A handout A voice recorder A videotape/DVD A microphone PowerPoint Preprogrammed communication device
Take a test	A review of test strategies A review of the information A practice test A double-spaced test Easy questions first A reader for the test A reduced number of choices by eliminating one or two choices In matching, a long column divided into smaller sections A computer As much time as needed An oral exam A performance-based test The option of drawing or labeling Simplified language
Complete worksheets	A word bank Clear directions File folder labels for students to stick answers onto Highlighted directions Fewer problems or questions Choice about type of writing instrument
Discuss	A talking object Note cards with students' ideas written on them Peer support A preprogrammed communication device with a question on it A piece of paper to draw ideas or concepts Choice about how to participate in the discussion The text the students are discussing A highlighted section of the text—have the student read and others discuss
Take notes	A lecture outline to complete during the lecture A chart A graphic organizer The teacher's notes from the day before An AlphaSmart Choice about how to take notes A copy of the teacher's notes with key words eliminated Lecture notes with pictures Photocopies or carbon copies from another student A laptop computer

(continued)

Table 7.4. *(continued)*

When the students are asked to	Consider providing students
Use a computer	A task card for how to start up the program Modified keyboard Enlarged font IntelliKeys An adjusted delay on the mouse An alphabetical keyboard Large keyboard Choice about what to work on
Read a text	Book on tape Larger print font Highlighter Choral reading Background information about the text Bullets of the main ideas Sticky notes to write questions on "Just-right books" Puppets Reading light Choice about what to read
Be organized	Color-coded folders A planner An agenda written on the board Assignments written on the board in the same place Assignments that are already three-hole punched A picture schedule A sticky note on desk of things to do A homework folder A desk check Clock or timer on desk A verbal rehearsal of the schedule A consistent routine
Write	Option to tell a friend his or her story before writing it A whole-group discussion Graphic organizers Use of bullet writing Pencil grips Option for student to dictate the story to an adult or a peer Words on a piece of paper that the student rewrites Stickers to fill in blanks Option to draw instead of write Raised-line paper—so students can feel lines

different students may have difficulty with each of these activities, for different reasons. The considerations listed on the right side of Table 7.4 have proved helpful for many students of all abilities.

ASSISTIVE TECHNOLOGY

Assistive technology is any type of technology that helps people with disabilities perform functions that might otherwise be difficult or impossible. The official definitions of assistive technology are as follows:

> Assistive technology in special education refers to any devices or services that are necessary for a child to benefit from special education or related services or to enable the child to be educated in the least restrictive environment. (IDEA 2004; 34 C.F.R. §300.308)

The term *assistive technology device* as outlined in IDEA 2004 means any item, piece of equipment, or product system, whether acquired commercially off the shelf, modified, or customized, that is used to increase, maintain or improve functional capabilities of children with disabilities. (PL 108-446, 20 U.S.C. §1401 [a][25])

The term *assistive technology service* means any service that directly assists a child with disabilities in the selection, acquisition, or use of an assistive technology device. The term includes:

- The evaluation of the needs of a child with a disability, including a functional evaluation of the child in the child's customary environment;

- Purchasing, leasing, or otherwise providing for the acquisition of assistive technology devices by children with disabilities;

- Selecting, designing, fitting, customizing, adapting, applying, maintaining, repairing, or replacing of assistive technology devices;

- Coordinating and using other therapies, interventions, or services with assistive technology devices, such as those associated with existing education and rehabilitation plans and programs;

- Training or technical assistance for a child with disabilities or, where appropriate, the family of a child with disabilities;

- Training or technical assistance for professionals (including individuals providing education or rehabilitation services), employers, or other individuals who provide services to, employ, or are otherwise substantially involved in the major life functions of individuals with disabilities. (PL 108-446, 20 U.S.C. §1401 [a][26])

Assistive technology includes mobility devices (e.g., walkers or wheelchairs), software, keyboards with large keys, software enabling students who are blind to use computers, or text telephones that enable students who are deaf to talk on telephones. A student who struggles with the fine motor skills involved with writing might use an AlphaSmart device, and a student who struggles to communicate might type his or her ideas into a computer, which then speaks the ideas aloud. If a student uses one type of assistive technology or another, you should learn as much as you can about the technology. If possible, ask for specific training on the technology so that you can assist the student in using the device, programming it, or fixing it if necessary. See the Chapter 7 Appendix for a list of useful web sites and resources for assistive technology.

TWENTY-ONE WAYS TO USE A STICKY NOTE

One SLP wrote a student a positive note on a sticky note every day. The student brought that note home and read it with his parents. The purpose of those notes was to provide only positive comments to the student. These kind notes really helped the student feel good about his performance at school. Sticky notes are amazingly versatile, especially when used to support students academically. Figure 7.3 shows 21 great ideas for using sticky notes.

COMMONLY ASKED QUESTIONS ABOUT ACADEMIC SUPPORT

Q.   What role do I play in supporting students who receive speech-language services when I am not in their classroom all day?

- As an individual agenda
- As a to-do list
- For a positive note in a pocket
- To mark page numbers
- As a reading guide
- To highlight sections of text
- To place under the directions
- To write questions to the students in their reading books
- As a written reminder about behavior
- As a way to monitor hand raising (every time the student raises a hand and answers, he or she marks the note)
- To cover up sections of a worksheet
- As a word bank (so students do not have to write but can, instead, place word in blank)
- For students who have a lot to say and blurt out a lot—have them write their questions on sticky notes and select one or two to ask
- To add ideas to a brainstormed list
- For students to give feedback to each other on projects or papers
- To label parts of a diagram
- To create a matching game
- To put students into groups
- For students to write questions or comments on and then to give to their teacher as a ticket out the door
- To ask a question to a peer, such as "Do you want to sit with me at lunch?"
- To summarize the main idea of a lesson, story, or activity

Figure 7.3. Twenty-one ways to use a sticky note.

A. Through indirect consultation, you can provide recommendations to the educational team about accommodations and modifications that support a student in the general education curriculum. You will not always have the role to implement your ideas. Yet, these recommendations are immensely beneficial to allow the student to benefit from special education and "specially designed instruction" under IDEA 2004.

Q. One student asks me to "go away" when I work with him. I cannot just let him sit there and fail. What should I do?

A. Listen to the student. If a student requests that you not work with him or her, do not support the student at that time. Instead, figure out how you might provide support without being physically next to the student. The lists in this chapter should be helpful to you.

Q. When a direction is given, a student calls my name and asks me to come and help. I am trying to fade my support, but the student will not do anything without me by her side. What should I do?

A. This student has become very dependent on adult support. We would suggest talking to the student about the need to try things by herself or about asking peers for help. Encourage all students in the class to use and provide help to one another. Involve your team in determining ways to increase the student's independence. Make sure the solutions will make the student feel empowered to become more independent—not punished for her dependence.

CONCLUSION

As an SLP, you provide both direct and indirect services in terms of the modifications, adaptations, assistive technology, or data collection procedures that are used. Both types of service delivery occur through purposeful planning for specific students. Your professional expertise, coupled with knowledge about the speech and language needs of each student, is very helpful for teams. It is essential that you provide teams with recommendations about accommodations and modifications that will support students during the academic portions of the day. The time that a teaching team spends discussing the types of academic support necessary to enable students to learn certain subjects or perform certain activities, how to fade support, and how to best adapt material and instruction across curricular areas is time well spent. It is interesting to note that, when teams make these changes for specific students, they can end up making improvements to teaching for all students. See the cartoon at the beginning of the chapter for an illustration of this concept. This chapter has focused on the many ways you can use strategies to support academics. The next chapter highlights behavioral support strategies.

NOTES

_____

_____

_____

_____

_____

_____

_____

_____

_____

_____

_____

_____

_____

_____

_____

_____

_____

_____

_____

_____

_____

_____

_____

7
Appendix

USEFUL WEB SITES AND
RESOURCES FOR ASSISTIVE TECHNOLOGY

AbleData
http://www.abledata.com

AccessIT: The National Center on Accessible Information Technology in Education
http://www.washington.edu/accessit/index.html

Alliance for Technology Access
http://www.ataccess.org

CAST: Transforming Education through Universal Design for Learning
http://www.cast.org

CATEA: Center for Assistive Technology and Environmental Access
http://www.assistivetech.net

National Center to Improve Practice in Special Education Through Technology,
  Media and Materials
http://www2.edc.org/NCIP

NATRI: National Assistive Technology Research Institute
http://natri.uky.edu

RehabTool
http://www.rehabtool.com/at.html

University of Connecticut Center for Students with Disabilities
http://www.csd.uconn.edu

8

Providing Behavioral Supports

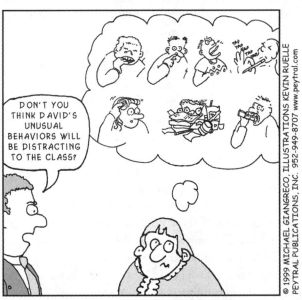

CONSIDERING HER STUDENTS WITHOUT DISABILITIES, MRS. BAKER REALIZES DAVID'S UNUSUAL BEHAVIORS AREN'T THAT UNUSUAL.

"With some of my students, behavior is a huge concern. I spend so much energy thinking of new ways to motivate and inspire students. It is really a big part of my job. Especially because when students can't communicate, they become frustrated, and frustration leads to behavior. This year alone, I have dealt with some significant behaviors."

—Carrie (SLP)

Julie once was giving a presentation to a large group of teachers. She asked them to list the most challenging behaviors they had seen among their students. The teachers thought about it for a while and then shared their lists with her as she wrote their ideas on chart paper. The lists included swearing, fighting, yelling, shutting down, becoming silent, running out of the room, hitting, and injuring oneself (e.g., biting one's own arm).

Julie then asked this same group of teachers whether they ever had participated in those behaviors themselves. She told them to raise their hands if they ever had sworn, fought, yelled, shut down, become silent, run out of a room, hit someone, or done anything to hurt themselves. The sound of nervous laughter filled the room as almost everyone raised their hands. This is no reflection about that particular group of professionals. Most people, on occasion, behave in ways that would be considered challenging or concerning. When Julie then asked the group to distinguish the students' challenging behaviors from their own behavior, one teacher responded, in a half-joking manner, "When I have bad behavior, I have a darn good reason!" Guess what? So do students.

Julie next asked the group to think about what they needed when they had engaged in bad behavior. They brainstormed this list: a hug, time away, someone to listen, a glass of wine, a nap, a cool-off period, changing the subject, talking to someone. Julie personally considers this a good list. Many of those things also help her calm down when she is angry or upset. Notice, however, not only what they suggested, but also what was not suggested. No teacher reported needing a sticker chart. No one said they needed to be lectured to or be removed from the room. Instead, like most people, these adults needed support, comfort, and calm, gentle understanding. Students need that, too.

In your job, you likely will work with students who have challenging behaviors. These may range from relatively nonconfrontational behaviors such as skipping class or shutting down to more significant or externalizing behaviors such as fighting with other classmates, running out of the school, or hurting oneself. This chapter begins with a discussion of typical responses to challenging behaviors and an overview of PBS. Then, we present a series of recommendations of what to do before, during, and after students demonstrate these types of challenging behaviors. At the end of the chapter, we answer some commonly asked questions.

THE TYPICAL RESPONSE TO CHALLENGING BEHAVIOR

Herb Lovett, a researcher who was at the Institute on Disability at the University of New Hampshire, described the typical response to challenging behavior:

Our initial response to an unwanted behavior is to react, to correct what we perceive to be unacceptable, inappropriate behavior. The thinking behind this perception is that the person exhibiting the behavior has lost control and that those who are in charge—in control—are responsible for regaining it through the application of methods and technologies specifically designed for this purpose. (1996, p. 136)

The major problem with this type of response is that, when the chosen method of control does not work, the teacher, therapist, or paraprofessional tends to become frustrated and, consequently, use more punitive methods for control. The intentions backfire, and, through a need to control and correct, teachers and therapists often create formidable barriers that further alienate them from those they are supposed to support and teach (Lovett, 1996). The way we think about behavior has a negative connotation: "What is wrong with this student?" as opposed to "How can I connect or support more effectively?" In Table 8.1 you will see a listing of new suggestions. What follows in this chapter are ideas and suggestions to move away from these typical responses to behavior toward a much more humanistic method of supporting students.

Table 8.1.   Give them what they need

For students who	Give them	For example
Talk a lot	More opportunity to talk	Talk walk, think pair share, debate, turn and talk
Move a lot	More opportunity to move	Stand and write, do graffiti-style work, write Michelangelo style, dance party, back to back
Want to lead	More opportunity to lead	Line leader, paper passer, helper, pointer
Appear shy	More support with social interactions	Write ideas before joining the group, clock partners
Are resistant	More choices	Choice of writing utensil, type or color of paper, types of manipulatives
Have tantrums	Time to calm down and then a plan when finished	"When you are ready, let's write down your first step."
Bully others	More opportunities to strengthen friendships	Tables at lunch based on interest, supported conversations with peers
Shut down	More ways to express frustration	"I need a break" card, a whiteboard to write feelings down
Make noise	Opportunities to make noise	A mouse pad to drum on, repetitive lines in read aloud
Interrupt	Opportunities to share during lessons	Turn and talk, say something, social break, cooperative learning groups
Have issues with assigned seating	Opportunities to select the best way to work	Use a clipboard on the floor, use a music stand, write Michelangelo style, do graffiti-style work

POSITIVE BEHAVIOR SUPPORT

PBS has been developed as a movement away from the traditional mechanistic, and even aversive behavior management practices that were being applied to students with disabilities. This approach "emphasizes the use of collaborative teaming and problem-solving processes to create supports that stress prevention and remediation of problem behaviors through the provision of effective educational programming and the creation of a supportive environment" (Janney & Snell, 2008, p. 2). The basic tenets of PBS are as follows:

1. Behavior is learned and can change.

2. Intervention is based on studying the behavior.

3. The intervention emphasizes prevention and teaching new behaviors.

4. Outcomes are personally and socially valued.

5. Intervention requires comprehensive, integrated supports. (Carr et al., 2002; Janney & Snell, 2008)

Note that PBS requires a team approach. You should not be expected to design a PBS program. Nevertheless, understanding the basic tenets of the program is important, because you likely will be responsible for helping to carry out behavior plans for some students.

PROACTIVE BEHAVIOR MANAGEMENT

Most challenging behavior can be avoided or managed by thinking ahead. Thinking ahead involves determining what works for the student.

··········

Gabe, a student with autism, has a very difficult time with changes in his schedule. He needs to know when transitions will occur. If he is surprised by a change in the schedule, he hides in his locker, paces, or runs around the room. One way to avoid this issue is to prepare Gabe for each day's schedule. The teaching team does this by having a peer greet Gabe's bus in the morning. Gabe and his peer then walk to the room together, and when they reach the classroom, they review the agenda for the day. Gabe also has an individual copy of the schedule in his planner. This strategy represents one of the most successful ways to prepare Gabe for the day ahead and to reduce his anxiety about the schedule.

··········

Building a Relationship

Lovett highlighted the importance of relationships and connections as more central than anything else related to supporting students behaviorally:

A positive approach [to behavior] invites people to enter into the same sort of relationship that most of us have and treasure: ongoing, with mutual affection and regard. In such relationships, we all make mistakes, are all in some ways inadequate and yet it is not the level of success that is the ongoing commitment. In the context of relationships, the success and failure of our work becomes harder to assess because the key elements no longer involve simply quantity but the more complex issues of quality. We professionals have routinely overlooked the significance of relationships. (1996, p. 137)

Getting to know your students and learning what they enjoy can be a truly helpful way to address challenging behaviors. "Creating a suitable level of rapport with students is an absolute essential prerequisite for helping students behave" (Knoster, 2008, p. 25).

• • • • • • • • • •

Mary, an SLP, believed she needed to get to know Dominique (a seventh-grade student) better in order to gain rapport and trust. Mary noticed that it was difficult to get to truly know Dominique in the inclusive classroom, so she held a "lunch bunch" for Dominique and six other students without disabilities from the inclusive classroom. They ate lunch together every Thursday in their seventh-grade classroom. Mary realized that it was not only an excellent way to get to know Dominique, but also a great way to support friendships and social interactions. Like Mary, SLPs often run lunch bunches in elementary school or lunch groups in middle and high school. This is a natural place for social communication to occur.

• • • • • • • • • •

One of the most important details of that anecdote is the way in which Mary created the lunch bunch. She approached the entire class about an opportunity to eat in the room each Thursday. She did not say it was a social group for Dominique but, instead, a "friendship group." Then she asked if anyone was interested. She was surprised to find that most of the class raised their hands, so she had students put names into a bucket. She then carefully selected the lunch bunch based on who might work well with Dominique. The students were unaware of the selection process. Mary realized that because of the interest level of the students and the success of Dominique's group, she could start another group. She began a Tuesday lunch bunch with another student on her caseload, and it is as successful as the first. She now provides her direct services to the second student during that lunch bunch time, while working on a variety of social and communication skills.

For SLPs, the kinds of goals that are easily worked into these groups include turn taking, articulation, social conversational skills, question asking, question answering, memory, executive functioning, attention, language syntax, voice volume, and pitch. There are many different ways to form relationships and to let students know that you trust them and that they can trust you. Some different methods include generally being there for the student if he or she needs you, having fun with the student, learning about the student's home life, making a home visit, seeing the same movies that the student enjoys, participating in the same activities the student likes, and talking to the student about his or her friends and hobbies. The next section discusses additional ways to build rapport each day with students.

How Do I Build Rapport with Students?

Latham (1999) provided steps for parents to build rapport with their children. These steps have been modified for therapists to use with students and are included here:

1. Demonstrate age-appropriate touch (high five, hand shake), facial expressions (reflect the nature of the situation), tone of voice (e.g., your voice also should match the situation), and body language (e.g., appear relaxed, keep your arms open, be attentive, look at the student).

2. Ask open-ended questions (e.g., "What are you doing after school?" "Tell me about that movie.").

3. Listen while the student is speaking. Ideally, talk less than the student (do not interrupt or change the subject).

4. Demonstrate the use of empathetic statements. Act like a mirror and reflect the child's feelings by expressing your understanding and caring.

5. Ignore nuisance behavior and let the little stuff slide.

Matching Instructional Practices to Student Strengths

One of the simplest ways to support students' positive behavior is to match instructional techniques to student strengths. For example, when a student who is a successful artist is allowed to draw his or her ideas during the social studies lecture, the student is more likely to be engaged and have positive behavior. As an SLP, you may not have control regarding how the instruction in the general education classroom is planned. However, some SLPs have very successfully helped teachers integrate new instructional techniques that support student learning. By trying out ideas and putting new plans in place, you can discover alternative approaches that others on the team also can try. You can always suggest new ideas. Never underestimate your power and creativity in supporting the students with whom you work.

· · · · · · · · · ·

Brent is a student with autism who shares in class frequently. He shares so frequently that it is sometimes a problem for the general education teacher. So, after speaking with Brent, he suggested using an idea marker. What that means is that he gets three sticky notes to "spend." They each represent one idea. He can share three times during any one class period. This technique became useful during each of Brent's courses. He puts one note down every time he shares. This creates a reminder for him about how many times he has shared. It worked so well during literature circle that each student in the small group also received three idea markers.

This solution not only helped Brent to choose wisely, but it also encouraged reluctant students and all of the students to share.

••••••••••

Knowing and understanding how students misbehave can help you identify what they need. Research has demonstrated that taking advantage of students' strengths can decrease negative behavior and increase on-task behaviors (Kornhaber, Fierros, & Veenema, 2004). See the following examples:

- If students are constantly moving or are bodily kinesthetic learners, they need more movement during instruction. For example, EunYoung needs to move during instruction. So, when the teacher reads aloud to the class, EunYoung is allowed to sit in a rocking chair. The teachers in EunYoung's class let the students sit however they like during certain class activities.

- If students are continually talking or are interpersonal learners, they need more interaction during learning. For example, Gwen works best when she is able to talk with peers. So, before writing a journal entry, she is given a few minutes to talk to a friend about what she plans to write.

- If students are constantly singing or are musically gifted, they need more music in school. Lucy enjoys music, so the teacher uses music during writing workshops. The music helps Lucy stay focused, and other students also enjoy it.

- If students enjoy making connections to their own lives or are intrapersonal learners, they need more time during school to make personal connections to the content. For example, Jerry enjoys making personal connections. So, during the *Little House on the Prairie* unit, Jerry's assignment is to determine how each of the settlers is like him and different from him.

- If students draw or doodle or are spatial learners, you can make art part of the learning process. For example, Rubin likes to draw. So, while he listens to a mini-lecture about cellular division, Rubin has the option of drawing the concepts.

- If a student enjoys mathematical calculations or is highly logical, you can use math and logic to strengthen the student's learning in other subjects. For example, Jorge loves math and struggles during English. So, the team has Jorge make Venn diagrams, time lines, and graphs about the characters in *Romeo and Juliet*. This helps him keep track of all of the characters, and, during discussion, he shares his charts with other students to help them remember the details of the book.

Set Up the Environment in a Way that Promotes Positive Behavior

One of the responsibilities of an SLP is to create an accessible learning environment. Have you ever walked into a classroom that felt controlled and stiff? Have you ever been in a learning environment that you wanted to escape from? What type of learning environment promotes learning? The following list offers ideas to help promote a more comfortable classroom environment:

- Arrange desks in a way that allows for easy student interaction. A circle of desks grouped into tables is more likely to promote interaction.

- Seat students with disabilities in different locations in the room. Do not group students with disabilities together.

- Create a calm, relaxed place in which students feel comfortable moving around and engaging with others.

- Create structure by posting the agenda or daily schedule.

- Add soft lighting to a corner area, so students can adjust lighting options.

- Add different types of seating (e.g., sit discs, arm chairs, rocking chairs).

- Do not isolate any student by seating him or her in a separate location.

- Make the classroom feel like a space for students by adorning the walls with student work.

- Have music playing softly in the background at times.

- If students are expected to sit on the floor, a soft, carpeted place will make them feel more comfortable.

- If a student struggles with personal space, have all students sit on carpet squares.

- If a student does not like to be called on in class without warning, set up a system to let the student know when the teacher will call on him or her.

Meet Students' Needs

All human beings require certain things to be happy and, therefore, well behaved. These things have been called *universal desires* (Lovett, 1996). Autonomy, relationships, interdependence, safety, trust, self-esteem, belonging, self-regulation, accomplishment, communication, pleasure, and joy are needs for all human beings. Helping students meet these needs is essential to creating learning environments in which students feel comfortable and safe; such feelings, in turn, help resolve behavioral issues.

Autonomy   *Autonomy* means the right or power to govern oneself or to be self-determined. To help students feel autonomous, provide choices and allow them to make as many decisions as possible. Examples include choice in seat location, whom to sit by, the materials to use for a project, the topic of a project, the type of writing instrument, whether to have something modified, and what to eat. Allowing students more choices enhances their ability to make decisions and become independent people.

Relationships and Interdependence   An entire chapter of this book (Chapter 6) has been dedicated to relationships. This is because relationships are deeply important. Students need to be allowed to have relationships and connections with their peers. Opportunities should be created for students to help one another. Chapter 6 suggests several strategies for facilitating relationships and building connections among students. When these needs are not met, students will invariably try to gain each other's attention. This bid for attention occurs in a variety of ways: it may be through hitting, tapping, or pestering. Students might also seem lonely and choose to sit by themselves. They may seem angry and try to get removed from certain settings through challenging behaviors.

Safety and Trust   Creating a safe, trusting relationship requires you to follow through when you say you are going to do something. Demonstrate that you can be trusted and that you are not there to punish or hurt any students. Keep your promises to students; "many people who engage in difficult behaviors have too much experience with broken promises" (Pitonyak, 2007, p. 18). Continually send the message that you are there to be trusted to help and support, not to punish and manage. Do not remove students from the learning environment. Every time a student is removed for a time-out or a brief stint in the hall, a clear message is sent to that student. The message is, "You are not welcome here. Your membership in this community is contingent on your behavior." This tends to create a vicious cycle: Students think that they do not belong, and they act in ways to demonstrate such thoughts; if they are removed, their suspicions are reinforced.

Pleasure and Joy   All students need pleasure and joy in their learning environments. When supporting a student, ask yourself, "How often does this student experience pleasure or joy in the classroom?" "How often does this student laugh or have fun with others?" "How can more time be devoted to pleasure and joy in the environment?"

Communication   All students deserve the right to communicate their needs and wants. Once, when Julie was observing students in a classroom, the teacher asked about the weather and date. One student using a communication device pushed a button to make the device say, "I know the answer." He pushed the button again and pushed it three more times during the morning meeting. He was never called on to answer. It seemed that the teacher was beginning to feel frustrated by the noise of the device, and eventually she walked over and took the device away from him. He later found the device and pushed the button to make the device say, "I feel sad." This story illustrates an important point. Communication is not something to be earned and taken away. Any attempt to communicate should be honored because all people need to be heard.

If students do not believe they are being heard, they will attempt to communicate their thoughts, feelings, and needs through their behavior. Students will assert their own independence, behave in certain ways to receive pleasure and joy, act out when they do not feel safe or need to communicate something, and act out simply to create more pleasure and joy in their lives. Purposefully creating such opportunities is essential to helping students avoid negative behavior. Students might be communicating something such as "I am lonely," "I do not feel safe," or "I do not know how to tell you what I need." The behavior they exhibit might not be easy to identify as communication, but it is important to remember that all behavior is communication. Part of the job of educators is trying to figure out what students are attempting to communicate in their behavior.

Ask Yourself: What Does This Person Need?

For each student, make a plan to help him or her receive more of the things that will fulfill his or her needs. For example, if you believe a student needs more choice, you should provide the student more choice.

We are aware that this recommendation contradicts most behavior systems and plans. Many people believe that if you give others what they need, they will just act out more. The opposite, however, is true. If you help meet students' needs, they will not need to misbehave more to get what they want (Kluth, 2003; Lovett, 1996; Pitonyak, 2007). See Table 8.2 for more ideas.

Here are some great questions to ask yourself:

- What might this person need?
- Does this person need more pleasure and joy in his or her school day?
- Does this person need more choice or control over what happens to him or her?
- Does this person need to feel more as if he or she belongs?
- Does this person need more relationships and interdependence?
- Does this person need more autonomy?
- Does this person need more access to communication?

First, determine each student's needs, and then work with your team to determine avenues to meet those needs.

Utilize Students as Problem Solvers

When a student becomes out of control, we often try to implement a behavioral management program that helps students comply with classroom rules. We do something to rectify the situation. Kohn argued, "Our responses to things we find disturbing, might be described as reflecting a philosophy of either doing things to students or working *with* them" (2006, p. 23). By working with students, teachers can transform their orientation to position students as expert problem solvers. This involves asking students what they need to be successful in a certain situation. Allow students to brainstorm solutions to problems, and implement their ideas.

Table 8.2. Asking new questions about behavior

Challenging behavior	Deficit thinking questions	New questions
Constantly moving	Why won't Zoey sit criss-cross during read-aloud time?	How can I restructure the read-aloud experience so Zoey can move and learn simultaneously?
Talking	Why is Liam interrupting during math when I am trying to teach a lesson?	How can I create interactive discussions during lessons, sending the message that meaningful participation is valued?
Singing	Why does Mia continue to hum during reading workshop when I've told her that this is an independent work time?	What sensory supports can I make available to Mia so that she is productive during reading workshop, but also does not distract others in our learning community?
All about me	Why does James continue to talk about activities and things he has done outside of school when we're exploring new science topics?	How can James share his background knowledge about science to motivate those around him? How can being a "science expert" support James' reading of nonfiction texts?
Shutting down	Why does Jazz hide her face when unfamiliar adults speak to her?	How can we support Jazz to develop relationships and interact effectively with new adults?
Asking why	Why does Ashley constantly challenge me by asking "why"?	What research opportunities can be built into learning experiences that allow Ashley to develop intricate knowledge about the "why" of concepts being studied?
Challenging or arguing	Why does Isaiah frequently bicker with classmates during playground time?	What social skills could to be taught to allow Isaiah to play and engage in cooperative learning groups effectively?
Running out	Why does Aiden scream and run out of the class?	Does Aiden have an effective communication system? What does this behavior communicate? Are the academic tasks differentiated to meet Aiden's needs?
Engaging in self-injurious behavior	Why does Chloe pick her fingers until they bleed and do other things that just hurt herself?	What is the function of this behavior? Did I ask Chloe why she does this?
Being rough with support staff	Why does Jack swat the paraprofessional when she is just trying to re-explain the directions?	Is the paraprofessional providing too much academic and social support in close proximity? How can we fade support? How can we teach Jack to ask for support when he needs it?

WEATHERING THE STORM

When confronting challenging behavior, school personnel often react by imposing consequences, threatening to impose consequences, removing rewards, or ignoring the behavior; in some instances, school personnel might force students to behave.

Forcing a student to behave might involve physically moving a student or providing hand-over-hand assistance.

Chelsea remembers observing one student engaging in difficult behavior in a classroom. The student was supposed to be working with two other students with some math manipulatives. The SLP was facilitating the cooperative group's conversation and problem solving skills. Instead, the student began running around and throwing the manipulatives at the SLP. The therapist responded by saying, "If you do not stop, I will write your name on the board, and you will not be able to work with your group anymore." The student did not stop. The SLP wrote the student's name on the board. The student continued running around. The therapist put a check mark next to the student's name as more manipulatives were thrown. She eventually said, "You are going to the time-out room!" She brought the student, kicking and screaming, to the time-out room, where he spent the remainder of the afternoon.

These types of situations are very difficult; you may have witnessed similar situations. There might not be easy solutions in these cases, but educators often jump to threats and isolation as their first line of defense. Researchers have determined that, although negative reinforcement may stop a behavior in the short term, it is not an effective or humane way to stop the behavior for the long term (Kohn, 2006).

We admit that it is easy for us to suggest alternatives; we were not the one who was frustrated by the behavior of the student who ran around throwing things at us. Nonetheless, consider some different reactions the therapist might have had. How do you think the interaction between the SLP and the boy throwing manipulatives might have changed had the therapist done any of the following?

- Walked over to the student and quietly asked, "What do you need right now?"
- Given the student a piece of paper and said, "Draw for me what is wrong."
- Calmly asked the student whether he needed a break or a drink of water.
- Asked the student to help clean up the mess.
- Given the student a responsibility: "Can you help me count the hot lunch sticks for the office?"
- Changed the activity entirely and asked the student to help her get ready for the next activity.
- Interpreted the student's behavior and said, "Are you finished?" or "Something seems wrong; can you help me understand what it is?"

Had the SLP responded with any of these reactions, it is doubtful that the student would have ended up in the time-out room with so much instructional time lost and at a major personal cost to the student and the SLP.

Alfie Kohn, a thoughtful researcher on rewards and punishments, suggested that rewards and punishments work in the short term. However, all educators need to ask themselves, "Work to do what?" and "At what cost?" When educators think big about what they want for their students in life, they might think they want all their students to be self-reliant, responsible, socially skilled, caring people. Rewards and punishments produce only temporary compliance. They buy obedience (Kohn, 2006). They do not help anybody develop an intrinsic sense of responsibility. In your own life, think of a task that you do not enjoy doing. For example, Julie personally dislikes taking out the garbage. Now, think for a moment: What if every time she took out the garbage, someone said to her, "Good job taking out the garbage, Julie"? Would that be more motivating? It wouldn't be for her. Sometimes, things people think are rewarding are actually not. It is also important to rethink providing rewards such as gum, candy, or stickers for "working hard." This reinforces the notion that what the student is doing is undesirable and needs a reward.

All Behavior Communicates Something

It is important to understand that all behavior communicates something. If a student is engaging in challenging behavior, ask yourself, "What might this student be communicating?" Once you have made your best guess at what the student needs, try to meet that student's needs. We watched a paraprofessional do this beautifully. A student, Hayden, was continually tapping a classmate, Sarah, on the back; the tapping seemed to bother Sarah. Instead of assuming that Hayden was trying to be obnoxious or to get attention, the paraprofessional interpreted Hayden's behavior as an attempt to interact with a friend. The paraprofessional whispered to Hayden, "Do you want to move closer and talk with Sarah? One way to start the conversation is to just say, 'Hi.'" Hayden moved closer and said, "Hi," and the conversation went on from there.

Some useful ways to interpret what a student is communicating include the following:

- *Ask him or her.* Say, "I see you are doing X; what do you want me to know?" or "It must mean something when you bang your head. What does it mean?"

- *Watch and learn.* Record everything the student does before and after a behavior. Meet with the team and try to determine what the student is attempting to gain from behaving this way.

- *Attribute positive motives.* One of the most important things is to consider what you believe about a particular child. Attribute the best possible motive consistent with the facts (Kohn, 2006). Assume that the student does not have malicious intent; the student probably is trying to get his or her needs met or to communicate something.

Every situation can be filtered through two different lenses. When you attribute the best possible motive consistent with the facts, you often see things in a positive and, possibly, more accurate light. This positive spin opens the door for more humanistic approaches to behavior. On the other hand, when behavior is interpreted as malicious or mean spirited, it is all too easy to respond in a similar way.

Have you ever been out of control? What do you need when you are out of control? Julie personally needs someone to listen, someone to talk to, someone to not give advice; sometimes, Julie needs a nap or some time away. When students are in the heat of the moment, they often need the most caring, from a calm person. They need an adult who is safe, calm, and cool and who will gently, calmly provide support.

What students do *not* need in the heat of the moment (or ever, for that matter) is to be ignored; to be yelled at; to be treated with hostility, sarcasm, or public humiliation; or to be forcefully removed from the situation.

Paula Kluth, an expert on behavior management (particularly with students who have autism), offered this advice:

> When a student is kicking, biting, banging her head, or screaming, she is most likely miserable, confused, scared or uncomfortable. The most effective and the most human response at this point is to offer support; to act in a comforting manner, and to help the person relax and feel safe. Teaching can come later. In a crisis, the educator must listen, support and simply be there. (2005, p. 2)

How Are the Other Students Behaving?

When students are supported by adults in the classroom, they invariably are under extra scrutiny. This sometimes leads to behavioral expectations that are more stringent for students with disabilities than for other students. In one case, we heard a teacher tell a student to sit up tall while working, although two other students in the room were sleeping and one other student was crawling on the floor. Observe how the other students are expected to behave; the student being supported should not be expected to perform at a higher behavioral standard. The cartoon at the beginning of this chapter illustrates this point.

Nothing Personal

As a special educator, Julie dealt with her fair share of challenging behaviors. The hardest thing was not to take anything personally. She had a student who was particularly good at figuring out her buttons and pushing them (or so she thought). The best advice she ever heard was to remember that the offensive behavior was "nothing personal." The students she supported invariably had challenging behavior. Whether she was working with them or not, they all were learning how to manage their own behavior. Sometimes, she would tell herself, "It is not personal. Even though this student has just called me a name, it is not about me right now." The challenging behaviors of some students are functions of their disabilities. Just as you would not get angry with a student who was having difficulty walking or reading—because you would assume that this was a function of the student's disability—you should not get angry with students who are struggling to behave. The best, most humane way to respond in these situations is to be helpful and supportive.

Think Like a Parent

Remember that every student is someone's child. When faced with a student's challenging behavior, imagine that you are someone who deeply loves the student. Try to imagine what it would be like if you had watched the child grow and learn from infancy onward; how would you react from that perspective? How might you react if it were your son, daughter, niece, or nephew? If you react from a position of love and acceptance, you are much more likely to respond with kindness and humanity than with punishment and control.

HELPING STUDENTS TO MOVE ON

If a student has just had a significant behavioral outburst, he or she may be embarrassed, tired, or still holding on to negative feelings. It is important to help students move past these experiences. After an outburst, you should let the student know that the crisis is over, validate his or her feelings, and help him or her move on. The phrases listed in Table 8.3 are offered as a guide to help you think about how you can talk to students to get them beyond emotional crises. The most important thing is for you to have a calm, loving tone in your voice as you communicate with the student.

Help the student repair any damage. When an adult makes a mistake or loses his or her temper, he or she first needs to repair the damage. Once, while giving a presentation, Julie made the mistake of using someone in the audience as an example. She did not think it would embarrass that person, but subsequently learned that it had. She felt awful; she had to repair the damage. She did so by writing a note of apology. Writing an apology note might not be the best way for a student to repair the damage after a behavioral outburst; the point is that you should help the student identify what might help fix the situation and involve him or her in repairing it. The solution should match the problem. For example, if a student knocks books off a shelf during a tantrum, the best solution is to have the student pick up the books. If a student rips up his artwork, the solution might be to have him either tape it together or create a new piece. If a

Table 8.3. How to communicate with a student after a behavior issue occurs

To communicate to a student	You might respond with
That the crisis is over	"You are done with that now." "The problem is done." Having the student draw the problem and then having him or her cross it out to signify that the situation has ended
That you validate this student's feelings	"It is okay to feel that way. I understand that was hard for you." "Now it is over." "I am sorry that was so hard for you." "I can tell you were really frustrated, angry, or upset." Drawing a picture of the student and then drawing thought bubbles over the student's head. Ask the student to help you identify what he or she was thinking and feeling.
That it is time to move on	"What do you need now?" "What can I help you with to get you back to work?" "Do you want to take a rest and prepare to get yourself back together?" "Would you prefer to get right back to work?" "Draw for me what you need right now."

student yells at a peer, a solution might be to have her write an apology note, draw an apology picture, or simply say, "I am sorry." You do not want to make the repair bigger than the problem. The main goal should be to get students back to work in a timely manner.

COMMONLY ASKED QUESTIONS ABOUT BEHAVIORAL SUPPORTS

Q.   If a student is not punished, will he or she not simply repeat the behavior?

A.   We do not believe in adding on a punishment. In fact, much research has been done on the use of time-outs and punishments. This research suggests that punishments work in the short term but have long-term negative effects on students (Kohn, 2006).

Q.   One of my students is not aggressive toward peers—only toward adults. What does that indicate?

A.   This type of aggression usually indicates a problem with the type or intensity of support being provided. Students often lash out at therapists, paraprofessionals, or teachers who make them feel different or uncomfortable because of the support being given. For example, Julie observed a 12-year-old girl who was being aggressive toward the paraprofessional. She noticed that the paraprofessional was providing intensive support by sitting next to the girl. The paraprofessional was also using a technique called "spidering" (crawling your hand up the back of the student's hair). The student seemed embarrassed and uncomfortable with that type and level of support. When the paraprofessional moved away from the student, the aggression stopped.

Q.   My team members want me to sit next to the student and provide direct support when I am in the classroom. I think there are better ways—what should I do?

A.   First communicate alternatives to the side-by-side support. Modify the work, change the writing utensil, give written prompts on a sticky note. You should provide the type and level of support that the team deems appropriate. However, if you think it is not helpful to the student, work with your team and discuss when it might be appropriate to fade your support: What would fading look like for this student? What other types of support can be in place to allow for student success?

Q.   Should a student leave the room if he or she is distracting other students?

A.   Leaving the room should be the absolute last resort. Try many different stay-put supports. Help the student stay in the environment for all of the reasons mentioned in this chapter. If a student leaves every time he or she makes a noise, that student learns that membership is contingent on being quiet or good. Of course you want to think about other students, but when inclusion is done well, all students understand that a certain student may make noise and that the student is working on that, just as other students may be working on other skills. Most students are surprisingly patient when given the chance and some information.

CONCLUSION

The way teams of educators plan for, support, and react to behavior is critical to student success. Remembering that all behavior communicates something and that all people need love and patience will help you be successful when supporting students. Supporting students who have challenging behavior is not easy; therefore, the next and last chapter of this book focuses on caring for yourself so that you can have the energy and ability to provide the best possible education for all students.

NOTES

9

Supporting You, Supporting Them

Self-Care

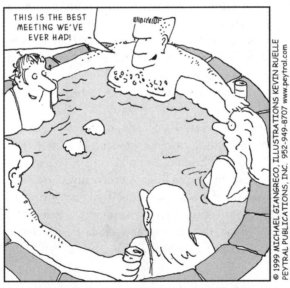

THIS IS THE BEST MEETING WE'VE EVER HAD!

TEAM MEMBERS FIND FUN WAYS TO
FACILITATE THEIR MEETINGS!

"Stopping to think about what I need to be successful as a person is something that I've gotten better at this year. I do my planning with colleagues before school, and after work I go straight to the gym for an hour. This is my calm and re-centering exercise. This is my uninterrupted time. Time that is reserved for me. This is what I need to do for myself to be a supportive, respectful therapist for my students. This is what I need to continue to nurture the relationships with my colleagues, and this is definitely what I need to go home to my family as a calm, loving, balanced momma!"

—Sara (SLP)

Julie finds herself a student of the process called *self-care*. She is continually seeking out ways to nurture herself. As a professor, author, consultant and, most important, mother of two small children, she often is in desperate and continual need of self-care. Consequently, she found this chapter the most difficult to write. In one memorable quest for self-care techniques, she helped put her kids to bed and soon found herself standing in the self-help aisle at the local bookstore with a close friend. She read different passages aloud. The books stated she should "become a bonsai tree" or imagine herself "on a glen surrounded by animals while breathing deeply." Her first thoughts were, "What is a glen?" and "What kind of animals?" "Are they dangerous?" "Are they rabid?" She and her friend began to laugh until other customers looked at them askance. Everyone takes care of himself or herself differently; every person needs to find the way that works best for him or her individually. This chapter does not provide you with a recipe for how to care for yourself; instead, it offers ideas or examples that may help you. Educators who are not rested, healthy, and reasonably content will have difficulty helping their students. Whether you deal with stress by running a marathon or by taking a bath, it is important to focus on what you enjoy and on what works to help you relieve stress and feel healthy and balanced.

The job of the SLP is not easy. Then again, no job worth doing is really easy. You may find the job quite rewarding or quite stressful, or it may vary from day to day. However, one thing is certain: You need to take care of yourself while taking care of others. In essence, you cannot give as fully to others if you are not meeting your own needs. You cannot help others solve problems if you are struggling with your own problems. You also need to set up your own support system. This chapter suggests strategies for problem solving, networking, and self-care. This chapter (and book) concludes with a new job description for SLPs.

PROBLEM SOLVING

Although you have read this book and have learned several ideas and strategies to handle many different kinds of problems or situations, problems inevitably will arise that you may not feel prepared to handle. When you come across a problem that you are having difficulty solving, consider the following general ideas or suggestions:

- Talk with other therapists or teachers in your school.
- Bring the problem to the special education teacher.
- Talk to another SLP.
- Talk to a PT.
- Sit down with the question: In what ways might I (fill in the problem here)? List all the potential solutions.
- Talk to the student.
- Talk with the principal.
- Talk to a parent.
- Talk with paraprofessionals.
- Draw the problem.
- Go for a walk—think only of solutions during the walk.
- Talk to your best friend or partner (keep all information about students confidential).

If meeting with others or brainstorming solutions by yourself does not help you discover a new solution, you may need a step-by-step problem-solving process, such as creative problem-solving (CPS).

CREATIVE PROBLEM-SOLVING PROCESS

The CPS process has a long history as a proven method for approaching and solving problems in innovative ways (Davis, 2004; Parnes, 1985, 1988, 1992, 1997). It is a tool that can help you redefine a problem, come up with creative ways to solve the problem, and then take action to solve it. Julie originally learned this method and used it as a teacher to solve problems with the students she supported. She continues to use this method to solve everyday personal and professional problems. Alex Osborn and Sidney Parnes (Osborn, 1993) conducted extensive research on the steps involved when people solve problems. They determined that people typically use a five-step process. Each step is described in the following list.

Explore the Problem

1. *Fact finding*—Describe what you know or perceive to be true about the challenge. Who? What? When? Where? How? What is true and not true about this problem?

2. *Problem finding*—Clarify the issue. View it in a different way. Finish this sentence: In what ways might we . . . ?

Generate Ideas

3. *Idea finding*—Generate as many ideas as possible; defer judgment and reinforcement (i.e., do not say things such as "good idea" or "that will not work," because then you would be passing judgment on the idea).

Prepare for Action

4. *Solution finding*—Compare the ideas against some criteria that you create. How will you know whether your solution will work? See Table 9.1 for sample criteria.

5. *Acceptance finding*—Create a step-by-step plan of action.

The following example describes how this process actually worked in solving a specific problem for a paraprofessional.

• • • • • • • • • •

A team working with Trevor, a first-grade boy, was having a difficult time getting Trevor off the playground at the end of recess. Trevor would run around and hide, and they could not

Table 9.1. The creative problem-solving process in action

Stage of creative problem-solving process	Examples from Trevor's team
1. Fact finding	It does not work to wait him out. It takes easily 10 minutes to get him off the playground. He does not respond to everyone leaving the playground—he continues to play. He enjoys playing tag with his friends. He has trouble with transitions. No one has ever asked him what he needs.
2. Problem finding	In what ways can we help Trevor return from recess promptly and happily?
3. Idea finding	Give him a time-out. Have him lose minutes off his recess time. Give him a timer or watch. Have a peer help him in. See how long he will play outside before coming in. Do not allow him to go outside for recess at all. Make a sticker chart. Give him extra recess.
4. Solution finding	We want this solution to . . . (example criteria) 1. Enhance the image of the student among peers. 2. Promote independence or interdependence. 3. Appeal to the student. 4. Increase and promote belonging. 5. Increase interaction with peers. 6. Seem logistically feasible.
5. Acceptance finding	The team finally decided on a solution for this problem, combining three ideas. They first met with Trevor to ask him what would help (they provided him with a menu of ideas); he decided on a timer with peer support. They gave Trevor a watch timer and asked him to identify a peer whom he was to find when the timer went off. When the timer rang (with 2 minutes remaining in recess), the two boys found each other and went to line up together. Problem solved.

Sources: Giangreco, Cloninger, Dennis, and Edelman (2002); Osborn (1993).

reach him or get him to go inside. The end of recess time was becoming a bit like a game of tag, except that the professionals definitely did not enjoy chasing Trevor around. Trevor would climb to the top of the slide, and if an adult came up, Trevor would slide down. If the adult went up the slide, Trevor would go down the monkey bars. This was almost humorous to watch unless you were members of the team, who felt frustrated and embarrassed. They considered the communicative intent of the behavior and decided that Trevor was likely trying to communicate that he did not want to come in from recess. Knowing that information, however, did not help the team identify what to do to get Trevor inside. They also knew that Trevor had a difficult time with transitions. The entire team sat together and engaged in a CPS process, which is briefly outlined in Table 9.1.

$$\cdots\cdots\cdots$$

BUILDING A NETWORK OF SUPPORT

"If you were all alone in the universe with no one to talk to, no one with which to share the beauty of the stars, to laugh with, to touch, what would be your purpose in life? It is other's life, it is love, which gives your life meaning. This is harmony. We must discover the joy of each other, the joy of challenge, the joy of growth."

—Mitsugi Saotome (1986, p. 1)

To sustain yourself as an SLP, you need a network of caring support. Do you feel isolated in your workplace? Do you believe that you could use more support? Think of all the people who love you and care about you. Now, consider others at work who also might feel isolated. In your school, classroom, or grade level, create a small team of support.

Create a Team of Support

One fourth-grade team created a support team by taking turns bringing in breakfast on Friday mornings. They ate together and talked, with no agenda. The conversations were fun and lighthearted, and the team members had time simply to connect with each other. Twice a year, they planned a Saturday morning breakfast to which they invited their families. As they ate together, they got to know more about each other and their loved ones. This helped to create a deeper sense of community for the professionals on the team.

Build a Community with Therapists

A group of SLPs, OTs, and PTs in one school district met after school every week to do yoga together. They then began running together. This time together helped them create a network of support, and they also got some exercise and fresh air while they talked.

Another group of SLPs met in the library and formed a book group that alternated between reading work-related books and books selected simply for pleasure. At the beginning of the year, they set their reading list. They organized themselves in such a way that they ended up convincing the director of special education to purchase the books through their professional development funds. For a useful set of work-related books and articles, see the lists in the Chapter 9 Appendix.

SELF-CARE

Have you ever been on an airplane and heard a flight attendant announce that if there is an emergency, you should place an oxygen mask on your own face before assisting your children? The idea behind that rule is that if the plane crashes, you want to make sure you are available to help the children. If you do not have oxygen, you will not be able to help them. In essence, that is what self-care involves: nurturing yourself outside of work so that you can be helpful and nurturing to the students you support.

Meet Your Own Basic Needs

Maslow (1999) identified the basic physiological needs of every human; these include oxygen, food, water, and regulated body temperature. Like any other human being, you need to make sure your needs are being met before you can help meet the needs of others. You might have to bring healthy snacks to school to keep yourself fueled for a long day at work. You might bring a water bottle with you so that you can stay hydrated throughout the day. You also might want to have a sweater with you or dress in layers; in many schools, temperatures frequently shift. Maslow's next level of need is safety and love. Surround yourself with loving people so that you feel loved and supported. Last, you need to get enough sleep every night. It is much more difficult to be prepared to support students if you are tired and cranky. These needs are at the very core of every person's physical and mental health.

Find an Outlet

Caring for yourself is critical to staying on the job and feeling balanced while doing it. Find ways to sustain yourself while outside of work. Consider physical outlets such as yoga, running, walking, biking, hiking, or swimming. Or, consider spiritual outlets such as meditation, prayer, or yoga to keep yourself spiritually balanced. The following is a simple exercise in meditation; try this exercise to help calm yourself down after a day or to prepare yourself before going into work.

An Exercise in Meditation

1. Find a comfortable place where you will not be bothered.

2. Sit with your eyes comfortably closed and turn your attention inward. Empty your mind of chattering thoughts. Relax.

3. If your mind begins to drift, gently return your focus inward.

4. Sit for as long as you feel comfortable.

5. When you are finished, answer these questions: How do you feel now? Are you energized, thoughtful, contemplative, relaxed, or anxious? Gently acknowledge those feelings and consider trying meditation another time.

Consider intellectual outlets such as playing games, reading, or writing. Or, try more creative outlets such as painting, sculpting, drawing, baking, cooking, scrapbooking, or generally creating something. Consider self-pampering activities such as taking baths, painting your nails, or getting massages. Employing these types of self-care strategies will help you feel balanced, healthy, and calm. See the Chapter 9 Appendix for a list of books on self-care.

As we have mentioned, we consider ourselves as learners, especially in the area of self-care. When working with children, you need to be constantly learning from them and for them. Our hope is that this book will be an impetus for your own learning. When reading this book, try out the strategies, and when you identify a strategy or idea that works, use it again. At the same time, remember that every context, every student, and every minute brings something new. It is important to reflect on when certain ideas or strategies work and how they work. The process is inevitably fluid. At the end of each day, ask yourself the following questions: 1) What worked today? 2) What did not work? and 3) What do I want to do differently tomorrow?

We conclude this book with a new job description for SLPs—a call to do things differently. We thank you for reading, and we wish you luck as you help the children you support to reach their full academic and social potential.

A SPEECH-LANGUAGE PATHOLOGIST'S JOB DESCRIPTION: WHAT YOUR STUDENTS MIGHT WANT YOU TO KNOW

Listen to me. Learn from me. Hear me. Support belonging. Be there, but give me space. Let me learn. Let me fail sometimes. Encourage independence. Always speak kindly. Ask, "What do you need?" Be safe. Handle me with care. Be respectful. Be gentle. Be trustworthy. Remember, I am a person first. If I am loud, be quiet. Encourage interdependence. If I am sad, wipe my tears. Help me connect with other students. Assume friendship is possible. Allow us to create together, laugh together, and have fun together. Assume competence always. Attribute the best possible motive consistent with the facts. Spark curiosity. Do not control. When I am happy, step back. Allow choice. Relax. Be a learner yourself. Ask, "How can I best help you?" Share positive stories with parents. Set me up to be successful. When I have difficulties, kindly redirect. Breathe. Step back. Speak softly. Encourage softly. Redirect softly. Follow my lead. Lead by loving. Give me space. Watch me thrive.

NOTES

9

Appendix

GREAT BOOK CLUB BOOKS FOR SPEECH-LANGUAGE PATHOLOGISTS

Armstrong, T. (1994) *Multiple intelligences in the classroom.* Alexandria, VA: Association for Supervision and Curriculum Development.

Blosser, J.L. (2012). *School programs in speech-language pathology: Organization and service delivery.* San Diego, CA: Plural Publishing.

Brendtro, L.K., Brokenleg, M., & Van Bockern, S. (2002). *Reclaiming youth at risk: Our hope for the future.* Bloomington, IN: National Educational Service.

Capper, C., & Frattura, E. (2008). *Meeting the needs of students of ALL abilities: How leaders go beyond inclusion.* Thousand Oaks, CA: Corwin.

Causton-Theoharis, J. (2009). *The paraprofessional's handbook for effective support in inclusive classrooms.* Baltimore, MD: Paul H. Brookes Publishing Co.

Frattura, E., & Capper, C. (2007). *Leading for social justice: Transforming schools for all learners.* Thousand Oaks, CA: Corwin.

Friend, M., & Cook, L. (2006). *Interactions: Collaboration skills for school professionals* (4th ed.). Boston, MA: Allyn & Bacon.

Giangreco, M.F., & Doyle, M.B. (Eds.). (2007). *Quick guide to inclusion: Ideas for educating students with disabilities* (2nd ed.). Baltimore, MD: Paul H. Brookes Publishing Co.

Gibbs, J. (2001). *Tribes: A new way of learning and being together.* Windsor, CA: CenterSource Systems.

Harmin, M. (1994). *Inspiring active learning.* Alexandria, VA: Association for Supervision and Curriculum Development.

Kliewer, C. (2008). *Seeing all kids as readers: A new vision for literacy in the inclusive early childhood classroom.* Baltimore, MD: Paul H. Brookes Publishing Co.

Kluth, P. (2010). *"You're going to love this kid!": Teaching students with autism in the inclusive classroom* (2nd ed.). Baltimore, MD: Paul H. Brookes Publishing Co.

Kluth, P. (2013). *"Don't we already do inclusion?": 100 ideas for improving inclusive schools.* Cambridge, WI: Cambridge Book Review Press.

Kluth, P., & Chandler-Olcott, K. (2008). *A land we can share: Teaching literacy to students with autism.* Baltimore, MD: Paul H. Brookes Publishing Co.

Kluth, P., & Danaher, S. (2010). *From tutor scripts to talking scripts: 100 ways to differentiate instruction in K–12 inclusive classrooms.* Baltimore, MD: Paul H. Brookes Publishing Co.

Kluth, P., & Schwarz, P. (2008). *"Just give him the whale!": 20 ways to use fascinations, areas of expertise, and strengths to support students with autism.* Baltimore, MD: Paul H. Brookes Publishing Co.

Kohn, A. (2006). *Beyond discipline: From compliance to community* (10th anniversary ed.). Alexandria, VA: Association for Supervision and Curriculum Development.

McCormick, L., Loeb, D.F., & Schiefelbusch, R. (2003). *Supporting children with communication difficulties in inclusive settings: School-based language intervention.* Boston, MA: Allyn & Bacon.

Montgomery, J.K. (2012). *Quick reference: Communication sciences and disorders.* Chippewa Falls, WI: Cognitive Press.

Nevin, A., Villa, R., & Thousand, R. (2009). *A guide to co-teaching with paraeducators: Practical tips for K–12 educators.* Thousand Oaks, CA: Corwin.

Paley, V.G. (1992). *You can't say you can't play.* Cambridge, MA: First Harvard University Press.

Ripley, K., Barrett, J., & Fleming, P. (2001). *Inclusion for children with speech and language impairments: Accessing the curriculum and promoting personal and social development.* New York, NY: David Fulton Publishers.

Rose, D.H., Meyer, A., & Hitchcock, C. (2005). *The universally designed classroom: Accessible curriculum and digital technologies.* Cambridge, MA: Harvard Education Press.

Sapon-Shevin, M. (2007). *Widening the circle: The power of inclusive classrooms.* Boston, MA: Beacon Press.

Scheurich, J.J., & Skrla, L. (2003). *Leadership for equity and excellence.* Thousand Oaks, CA: Corwin.

Schon, D.A. (1983). *The reflective practitioner. How professionals think in action.* New York, NY: Basic Books.

Schraeder, T. (2013). *A guide to school services in speech-language pathology.* San Diego, CA: Plural Publishing.

Schwarz, P., & Kluth, P. (2008). *You're welcome: 30 innovative ideas for the inclusive classroom.* Portsmouth, NH: Heinemann.

Silberman, M. (1996). *Active learning: 101 strategies to teach any subject.* Boston, MA: Allyn & Bacon.

Snell, M., & Janney, R. (2005). *Teacher's guides to inclusive practices: Collaborative teaming* (2nd ed.). Baltimore, MD: Paul H. Brookes Publishing Co.

Stainback, S., & Stainback, W. (1996). *Inclusion: A guide for educators.* Baltimore, MD: Paul H. Brookes Publishing Co.

Tashie, C., Shapiro-Barnard, S., & Rossetti, Z. (2006). *Seeing the charade: What people need to do and undo to make friendships happen.* Nottingham, United Kingdom: Inclusive Solutions.

Theoharis, G. (2009). *The school leaders our children deserve: 7 keys to equity, social justice, and school reform.* New York, NY: Teachers College Press.

Thousand, J., Villa, R., & Nevin, A. (2007). *Differentiating instruction: Collaborative planning and teaching for universally designed learning.* Thousand Oaks, CA: Corwin.

Tomlinson, C.A. (2004). *How to differentiate instruction in the mixed ability classroom* (2nd ed.). Alexandria, VA: Association for Supervision and Curriculum Development.

Udvari-Solner, A., & Kluth, P. (2008). *Joyful learning: Active and collaborative learning in the inclusive classroom.* Thousand Oaks, CA: Corwin.

Villa, R.A., & Thousand, J.S. (Eds.). (2005). *Creating an inclusive school* (2nd ed.). Alexandria, VA: Association for Supervision and Curriculum Development.

Villa, R.A., Thousand, J.S., & Nevin, A.I. (2010). *Collaborating with students in instruction and decision making: The untapped resource.* Thousand Oaks, CA: Corwin.

Wheatley, M. (2002). *Turning to one another: Simple conversations to restore hope to the future.* San Francisco, CA: Berrett-Koehler.

GREAT ARTICLES FOR SPEECH-LANGUAGE PATHOLOGISTS

Causton-Theoharis, J. (2009). The golden rule of supporting in inclusive classrooms: Support others as you would wish to be supported. *Teaching Exceptional Children, 42*(2), 36–43.

Causton-Theoharis, J., & Malmgren, K. (2005). Building bridges: Strategies to help paraprofessionals promote peer interactions. *Teaching Exceptional Children, 37*(6), 18–24.

Causton-Theoharis, J., & Theoharis, G. (2008, September). Creating inclusive schools for ALL students. *The School Administrator, 65*(8), 24–30.

Ehren, B.J. (2000). Maintaining a therapeutic focus and sharing responsibility for student success: Keys to in-classroom speech-language services. *American Speech-Language-Hearing Association, 31,* 219–229.

Giangreco, M.F. (2004). "The stairs didn't go anywhere!": A self-advocate's reflections on specialized services and their impact on people with disabilities. In M. Nid, J. Rix, K. Sheehy, & K. Simmons (Eds.), *Inclusive education: diverse perspectives* (pp. 32–42). London, United Kingdom: David Fulton Publishers.

Kluth, P., Villa, R.A., & Thousand, J.S. (2001). "Our school doesn't offer inclusion" and other legal blunders. *Educational Leadership, 59,* 24–27.

McLesky, J., & Waldron, N. (2002). School change and inclusive schools: Lesson learned from practice. *Phi Delta Kappan, 84*(1), 65–72.

Riehl, C.J. (2000). The principal's role in creating inclusive schools for diverse students: A review of normative, empirical, and critical literature on the practice of educational administration. *Review of Educational Research, 70*(1), 55–81.

SELF-CARE BOOKS

Byrne, R. (2006). *The secret.* New York, NY: Atria Books/Beyond Words.

Carlson, R. (1998). *Don't sweat the small stuff at work: Simple ways to minimize stress and conflict while bringing out the best in yourself and others.* New York, NY: Hyperion.

Covey, S.R. (2004). *The 7 habits of highly effective people: Powerful lessons in personal change* (15th anniversary ed.). New York, NY: Free Press.

Fontana, D. (1999). *Learn to meditate: A practical guide to self-discovery.* London, United Kingdom: Duncan Baird.

Hoff, B. (1983). *The tao of Pooh.* New York, NY: Penguin.

Moran, V. (1999). *Creating a charmed life: Sensible, spiritual secrets every busy woman should know.* New York, NY: HarperOne.

Palmer, P. (1999). *Let your life speak: Listening to the voice of vocation.* San Francisco, CA: Jossey-Bass.

Palmer, P. (2004). *A hidden wholeness: The journey towards the undivided life.* San Francisco, CA: Jossey-Bass.

Reynolds, S. (2005). *Better than chocolate.* Berkeley, CA: Ten Speed Press.

SARK. (1991). *A creative companion: How to free your creative spirit.* New York, NY: Fireside.

SARK. (1994). *Living juicy: Daily morsels for your creative soul.* New York, NY: Fireside.

SARK. (1997). *Succulent wild women.* New York, NY: Fireside.

SARK. (2005). *Make your creative dreams real: A plan for procrastinators, perfectionists, busy people, and people who would really rather sleep all day.* New York, NY: Fireside.

Topchik, G. (2001). *Managing workplace negativity.* New York, NY: AMACOM.

Wheatley, M.J. (2002). *Turning to one another: Simple conversation to restore hope in the future.* San Francisco, CA: Berrett-Koehler Press.

References

American Psychiatric Association. (2000). *Diagnostic and statistical manual of mental disorders* (4th ed., text revision). Washington, DC: Author.

American Speech-Language-Hearing Association. (1996). *Inclusive practices for children and youths with communication disorders* [Technical Report]. Available from www.asha.org/policy

American Speech-Language-Hearing Association. (2002a). *A workload analysis approach for establishing speech-language caseload standards in the schools* [guidelines]. Retrieved from www.asha.org/policy

American Speech-Language-Hearing Association. (2002b). *A workload analysis approach for establishing speech-language caseload standards in the schools* [technical report]. Retrieved from www.asha.org/policy

American Speech-Language-Hearing Association. (2007) *Scope of practice in speech-language pathology* [scope of practice]. Retrieved from http://www.asha.org/policy/SP2007–00283.htm

American Speech-Language-Hearing Association. (2010). *Roles and responsibilities of speech-language pathologists in schools* [professional issues statement]. Retrieved from http://www.asha.org/policy/PI2010–00317.htm

American Speech-Language-Hearing Association. (2013). *The history of speech and language therapists.* Retrieved from http://www.asha.org/about/history/

Armstrong, T. (1994). *Multiple intelligences in the classroom.* Alexandria, VA: Association for Supervision and Curriculum Development.

Armstrong, T. (2000a). *In their own way: Discovering and encouraging your child's multiple intelligences.* New York, NY: Jeremy P. Tarcher, Penguin Group (USA) LLC.

Armstrong, T. (2000b). *Multiple intelligences in the classroom.* Alexandria, VA: Association for Supervision and Curriculum Development.

Ashby, C.E. (2008). *"Cast into a cold pool": Inclusion and access in middle school for students with labels of mental retardation and autism* (Unpublished doctoral dissertation). Syracuse University, Syracuse, NY.

Biklen, D. (2005). *Autism and the myth of the person alone* (pp. 80–82). New York: New York University Press.

Biklen, D., & Burke, J. (2006). Presuming competence. *Equity & Excellence in Education, 39,* 166–175.

Blatt, B. (1987). *The conquest of mental retardation.* Austin, TX: PRO-ED.

Blosser, J.L. (2012). *School programs in speech-language pathology: Organization and service delivery.* San Diego, CA: Plural Publishing.

Bonner Foundation. (2008). Conflict resolution: Steps for handling interpersonal dynamics. In *Bonner civic engagement training modules.* Retrieved from http://bonnernetwork.pbworks.com/w/page/13112080/Bonner%20Training%20Modules%20%28with%20Descriptions%29

Brendtro, L.K., Brokenleg, M., & Van Bockern, S. (2002). *Reclaiming youth at risk: Our hope for the future.* Bloomington, IN: National Educational Service.

Byrne, R. (2006). *The secret*. New York, NY: Atria Books/Beyond Words.

Callahan, C. (1997). *Advice about being an LD student*. Retrieved from http://www.ldonline.org/firstperson/8550

Capper, C., & Frattura, E. (2008). *Meeting the needs of students of ALL abilities: How leaders go beyond inclusion*. Thousand Oaks, CA: Corwin.

Carlson, R. (1998). *Don't sweat the small stuff at work: Simple ways to minimize stress and conflict while bringing out the best in yourself and others*. New York, NY: Hyperion.

Carr, E.G., Dunlap, G., Horner, R.H., Koegel, R.L., Turnbull, A., Sailor, W., . . ., Fox, L. (2002). Positive behavior support: Evolution of an applied science. *Journal of Positive Behavior Interventions, 4*(1), 4–16.

Casey, K., & Vanceburg, M. (1996). *A promise of a new day: A book of daily meditations*. Center City, MN: Hazelden.

Causton-Theoharis, J. (2003) *Increasing interactions between students with disabilities and their peers via paraprofessional training*, Unpublished doctoral dissertation. University of Wisconsin–Madison.

Causton-Theoharis, J. (2009a). The golden rule of supporting in inclusive classrooms: Support others as you would wish to be supported. *Teaching Exceptional Children, 42*(2), 36–43.

Causton-Theoharis, J. (2009b). *The paraprofessional's handbook for effective support in inclusive classrooms*. Baltimore, MD: Paul H. Brookes Publishing Co.

Causton-Theoharis, J., & Malmgren, K. (2005). Building bridges: Strategies to help paraprofessionals promote peer interactions. *Teaching Exceptional Children, 37*(6), 18–24.

Causton-Theoharis, J., & Theoharis, G. (2008, September). Creating inclusive schools for all students. *The School Administrator, 65*(8), 24–30.

Covey, S.R. (2004). *The 7 habits of highly effective people: Powerful lessons in personal change* (15th anniversary ed.). New York, NY: Free Press.

Crossley, R. (2013, July). *Defending the right to communicate*. Presentation at the ICI Summer Institute, Syracuse University, NY.

Data Accountability Center. [n.d.]. *Individuals with Disabilities Education Act [IDEA] data*. Retrieved December 1, 2008, from http://www.ideadata.org/docs/PartBTrendData/B2A.html

Davis, G. (2004). *Creativity is forever* (5th ed.). Dubuque, IA: Kendall Hunt.

Donnellan, A. (1984). The criterion of the least dangerous assumption. *Behavioral Disorders, 9*, 141–150.

Doyle, M.B. (2008). *The paraprofessional's guide to the inclusive classroom: Working as a team* (3rd ed.). Baltimore, MD: Paul H. Brookes Publishing Co.

Dunn, W. (1990). A comparison of service provision models in school-based occupational therapy services: A pilot study. *Occupational Therapy Journal of Research, 10*, 300–320.

Education for All Handicapped Children Act of 1975, PL 94-142, 20 U.S.C. §§ 1400 *et seq.*

Ehren, B.J. (2000). Maintaining a therapeutic focus and sharing responsibility for student success: Keys to in-classroom speech-language services. *American Speech-Language-Hearing Association, 31*, 219–229.

Ehren, B., Montgomery, J., Rudebusch, J., & Whitmire, K. (2013). Responsiveness to intervention: New roles for speech-language pathologists. *American Speech-Language-Hearing Association*. Retrieved from http://www.asha.org/SLP/schools/prof-consult/NewRolesSLP/

FAS Community Resource Center. (2008). *Information about fetal alcohol syndrome (FAS) and fetal alcohol spectrum disorders (FASD)*. Retrieved from http://www.come-over.to/FASCRC

Fontana, D. (1999). *Learn to meditate: A practical guide to self-discovery*. London, United Kingdom: Duncan Baird.

Frattura, E., & Capper, C. (2007). *Leading for social justice: Transforming schools for all learners*. Thousand Oaks, CA: Corwin.

Friend, M., & Cook, L. (2006). *Interactions: Collaboration skills for school professionals* (4th ed.). Boston, MA: Allyn & Bacon.

Friend, M., & Reising, M. (1993, Summer). Co-teaching: An overview of the past, a glimpse at the present, and considerations for the future. *Preventing School Failure, 37*(4), 6–10.

Gabel, A. (2006). Stop asking me if I need help. In E.B. Keefe, V.M. Moore, & F.R. Duff (Eds.), *Listening to the experts: Students with disabilities speak out* (pp. 35–40). Baltimore, MD: Paul H. Brookes Publishing Co.

Gardner, H. (1993). *Frames of mind: A theory of multiple intelligences*. New York, NY: Basic Books.

Giangreco, M.F. (2004). "The stairs didn't go anywhere!": A self-advocate's reflections on specialized services and their impact on people with disabilities. In M. Nid, J. Rix, K. Sheehy, & K. Simmons (Eds.),

Inclusive education: diverse perspectives (pp. 32–42). London: David Fulton Publishers in association with The Open University. Thousands Oaks, CA: Crown Press. (Reprinted from Giangreco, M.F. [1996]. "The stairs didn't go anywhere!": A self-advocate's reflections on specialized services and their impact on people with disabilities. *Physical Disabilities: Education and Related Services, 14*[2], 1–12.)

Giangreco, M.F. (2007). *Absurdities and realities of special education: The complete digital set.* [CD]. Thousand Oaks, CA: Corwin.

Giangreco, M.F., Cloninger, C.J., Dennis, R., & Edelman, S.W. (2002). Problem-solving methods to facilitate inclusive education. In J.S. Thousand, R.A. Villa, & A.I. Nevin (Eds.), *Creativity and collaborative learning: The practical guide to empowering students, teachers, and families* (2nd ed., pp. 111–134). Baltimore, MD: Paul H. Brookes Publishing Co.

Giangreco, M.F., & Doyle, M.B. (Eds.). (2007). *Quick-guides to inclusion: Ideas for educating students with disabilities* (2nd ed.). Baltimore, MD: Paul H. Brookes Publishing Co.

Giangreco, M.F., Edelman, S.W., Luiselli, E.T., & MacFarland, S.Z. (1997). Helping or hovering: The effects of paraprofessional proximity on students with disabilities. *Exceptional Children, 64*(1), 7–18.

Gibbs, J. (2001). *Tribes: A new way of learning and being together.* Windsor, CA: CenterSource Systems.

Gray, C. (2013). *The Gray center.* Retrieved July 15, 2013, from https://www.thegraycenter.org/social -stories/carol-gray

Harmin, M. (1994). *Inspiring active learning.* Alexandria, VA: Association for Supervision and Curriculum Development.

Hoff, B. (1983). *The tao of Pooh.* New York, NY: Penguin.

Huefner, D.S. (2000). *Getting comfortable with special education law: A framework for working with children with disabilities.* Norwood, MA: Christopher-Gordon.

Individuals with Disabilities Education Improvement Act (IDEA) of 2004, PL 108-446, 20 U.S.C. §§ 1400 *et seq.*

Information on bipolar and other mental health disorders. (n.d.) *Borderline personality disorder.* Retrieved from http://www.angelfire.com/home/bphoenix1/border.html

Institut Pasteur. (n.d.). *Louis Pasteur's biography.* Retrieved from http://www.pasteur.fr/ip/easysite/ pasteur/fr/institut-pasteur/histoire/biographie-de-louis-pasteur#

Janney, R., & Snell, M.E. (2004). *Teachers' guides to inclusive practices: Modifying schoolwork* (2nd ed.). Baltimore, MD: Paul H. Brookes Publishing Co.

Janney, R., & Snell, M.E. (2008). *Teachers' guides to inclusive practices: Behavioral support* (2nd ed.). Baltimore, MD: Paul H. Brookes Publishing Co.

Jones, R.C. (1998–2006). *Strategies for reading comprehension: Clock buddies.* Retrieved from http:// www.readingquest.org/strat/clock_buddies.html

Kasa, C., & Causton-Theoharis, J. (n.d.) *Strategies for success: Creating inclusive classrooms that work* (pp. 16–17). Pittsburgh, PA: The PEAL Center. Retrieved from http://wsm.ezsitedesigner.com/share/ scrapbook/47/472535/PEAL-S4Success_20pg_web_version.pdf

Kasa-Hendrickson, C., & Buswell, W. (2007). *Strategies for presuming competence.* Unpublished handout.

Keller, H. (1903). *The story of my life.* New York, NY: Doubleday, Page.

Kliewer, C. (2008). *Seeing all kids as readers: A new vision for literacy in the inclusive early childhood classroom.* Baltimore, MD: Paul H. Brookes Publishing Co.

Kliewer, C., & Biklen, D. (1996). Labeling: Who wants to be called retarded? In W. Stainback & S. Stainback (Eds.), *Controversial issues confronting special education: Divergent perspectives* (2nd ed., pp. 83–111). Boston, MA: Allyn & Bacon.

Kluth, P. (2003). *"You're going to love this kid!": Teaching students with autism in the inclusive classroom.* Baltimore, MD: Paul H. Brookes Publishing Co.

Kluth, P. (2005). Calm in crisis. Adapted from P. Kluth (2003), *"You're going to love this kid!": Teaching students with autism in the inclusive classroom.* Baltimore, MD: Paul H. Brookes Publishing Co. Retrieved from http://www.paulakluth.com/readings/autism/calm-in-crisis/

Kluth, P. (2010). *"You're going to love this kid!": Teaching students with autism in the inclusive classroom* (2nd ed.). Baltimore, MD: Paul H. Brookes Publishing Co.

Kluth, P. (2013). *"Don't we already do inclusion?": 100 ideas for improving inclusive schools.* Cambridge, WI: Cambridge Book Review Press.

Kluth, P., & Chandler-Olcott, K. (2008). *A land we can share: Teaching literacy to students with autism.* Baltimore, MD: Paul H. Brookes Publishing Co.

Kluth, P., & Danaher, S. (2010). *From tutor scripts to talking scripts: 100 ways to differentiate instruction in K–12 inclusive classrooms.* Baltimore, MD: Paul H. Brookes Publishing Co.

Kluth, P., & Schwarz, P. (2008). *"Just give him the whale!": 20 ways to use fascinations, areas of expertise, and strengths to support students with autism.* Baltimore, MD: Paul H. Brookes Publishing Co.

Kluth, P., Villa, R.A., & Thousand, J.S. (2001). "Our school doesn't offer inclusion" and other legal blunders. *Educational Leadership, 59,* 24–27.

Knoster, T.P. (2008). *The teacher's pocket guide for effective classroom management.* Baltimore, MD: Paul H. Brookes Publishing Co.

Kohn, A. (2006). *Beyond discipline: From compliance to community* (10th anniversary ed.). Alexandria, VA: Association for Supervision and Curriculum Development.

Kornhaber, M., Fierros, E., & Veenema, S. (2004). *Multiple intelligences: Best ideas from research and practice.* Boston, MA: Pearson Education.

Kunc, N. (1992). The need to belong: Rediscovering Maslow's hierarchy of needs. In R. Villa, J. Thousand, W. Stainback, & S. Stainback (Eds.), *Restructuring for caring and effective education* (pp. 21–40). Baltimore, MD: Paul H. Brookes Publishing Co.

Kunc, N., & Van der Klift, E. (1996). *A credo for support.* Vancouver, British Columbia: The BroadReach Centre.

Latham, G.I. (1999). *Parenting with love: Making a difference in a day.* Logan, UT: P&T Ink.

Lovett, H. (1996). *Learning to listen: Positive approaches and people with difficult behavior.* Baltimore, MD: Paul H. Brookes Publishing Co.

Malmgren, K.W., & Causton-Theoharis, J.N. (2006). Boy in the bubble: Effects of paraprofessional proximity and other pedagogical decisions on the interactions of a student with behavioral disorders. *Journal of Research in Childhood Education, 20*(4), 301–312.

Maslow, A.H. (1999). *Toward a psychology of being.* New York, NY: John Wiley & Sons.

Mavis. (2003, October 7). *Living in the hearing and deaf worlds.* Retrieved from http://www.raisingdeafkids.org/meet/deaf/mavis/worlds.php

McCormick, L., Loeb, D.F., & Schiefelbusch, R. (2003). *Supporting children with communication difficulties in inclusive settings: School-based language intervention.* Boston, MA: Allyn & Bacon.

McLesky, J., & Waldron, N. (2002). School change and inclusive schools: Lessons learned from practice. *Phi Delta Kappan, 84*(1), 65–72.

McLeskey, J., & Waldron, N. (2006). Comprehensive school reform and inclusive schools: Improving schools for all students. *Theory into Practice, 45*(3), 269–278.

Molton, K. (2000). *Dispelling some myths about autism.* Retrieved from http://www.nas.org.uk/nas/jsp/polopoly.jsp?d=120&a=2202

Montgomery, J.K. (2012). *Quick reference: Communication sciences and disorders.* Chippewa Falls, WI: Cognitive Press.

Mooney, J. (2007). *The short bus: A journey beyond normal.* New York, NY: Henry Holt and Company, LLC.

Moran, V. (1999). *Creating a charmed life: Sensible, spiritual secrets every busy woman should know.* New York, NY: HarperOne.

Mueller, P.H. (2002). The paraeducator paradox. *Exceptional Parent, 32*(9), 64–67.

Murawski, W.W., & Dieker, L.A. (2004). Tips and strategies for co-teaching at the secondary level. *Teaching Exceptional Children, 36*(5), 52–58.

National Association of School Psychologists. (2000). *What is a school psychologist?* Retrieved from http://www.nasponline.org/about_sp/whatis.aspx

Nevin, A., Villa, R., & Thousand, R. (2009). *A guide to co-teaching with paraeducators: Practical tips for K–12 educators.* Thousand Oaks, CA: Corwin.

No Child Left Behind Act of 2001, PL 107-110, 115 Stat. 1425, 20 U.S.C. §§ 6301 *et seq.*

Orwell, G. (1946). Politics and the English language. *Horizon, 13*(76), 252–265. Retrieved from https://www.mtholyoke.edu/acad/intrel/orwell46.htm

Osborn, A.F. (1993). *Applied imagination: Principles and procedures of creative problem-solving* (3rd rev. ed.). Buffalo, NY: Creative Education Foundation Press.

Paley, V.G. (1992). *You can't say you can't play.* Cambridge, MA: First Harvard University Press.

Palmer, P. (1999). *Let your life speak: Listening to the voice of vocation.* San Francisco, CA: Jossey-Bass.

Palmer, P. (2004). *A hidden wholeness: The journey towards the undivided life.* San Francisco, CA: Jossey-Bass.

Parker, K. (2008). *Meet RhapsodyBlue.* Retrieved from http://www.angelfire.com/country/rhapsodyblue22/page2.html

Parnes, S.J. (1985). *A facilitating style of leadership.* Buffalo, NY: Bearly.

Parnes, S.J. (1988). *Visionizing: State-of-the-art processes for encouraging innovative excellence.* East Aurora, NY: D.O.K.

Parnes, S.J. (Ed.). (1992). *Source book for creative problem solving: A fifty-year digest of proven innovation processes.* Buffalo, NY: Creative Education Foundation Press.

Parnes, S.J. (1997). *Optimize the magic of your mind.* Buffalo, NY: Creative Education Foundation Press.

Paul-Brown, D., & Diggs, M.C. (1993, Winter). Recognizing and treating speech and language disabilities. *American Rehabilitation, 19* (4), 30.

PEAK Parent Center. (n.d.). *Accommodations and modifications fact sheet.* Retrieved from http://www .peatc.org/peakaccom.htm

Peterson, J.M., & Hittie, M.M. (2002). *Inclusive teaching: Creating effective schools for all learners.* Boston, MA: Allyn & Bacon.

Pitonyak, D. (2007). *The importance of belonging.* Retrieved from http://www.dimagine.com/page5.html

Reynolds, S. (2005). *Better than chocolate.* Berkeley, CA: Ten Speed Press.

Riehl, C.J. (2000). The principal's role in creating inclusive schools for diverse students: A review of normative, empirical, and critical literature on the practice of educational administration. *Review of Educational Research, 70*(1), 55–81.

Ripley, K., Barrett, J., & Fleming, P. (2001). *Inclusion for children with speech and language impairments: Accessing the curriculum and promoting personal and social development.* New York, NY: David Fulton Publishers.

Rosa's Law, 2010, PL 111-256, 20 U.S.C. §§ 1400 *et seq.*

Rose, D.H., Meyer, A., & Hitchcock, C. (2005). *The universally designed classroom: Accessible curriculum and digital technologies.* Cambridge, MA: Harvard Education Press.

Rubin, S. (2003, December). *Making dreams come true.* Paper presented at the annual conference of TASH, Chicago, IL.

Saotome, M. (1986). The dojo: Spiritual oasis. In *Aikido and the harmony of nature* (pp. 246–248). Boulogne, France: SEDIREP.

Sapon-Shevin, M. (2007). *Widening the circle: The power of inclusive classrooms.* Boston, MA: Beacon Press.

SARK. (1991). *A creative companion: How to free your creative spirit.* New York, NY: Fireside.

SARK. (1994). *Living juicy: Daily morsels for your creative soul.* New York, NY: Fireside.

SARK. (1997). *Succulent wild women.* New York, NY: Fireside.

SARK. (2005). *Make your creative dreams real: A plan for procrastinators, perfectionists, busy people, and people who would really rather sleep all day.* New York, NY: Fireside.

Schalock, R.L., & Braddock, D.L. (2002). *Out of the darkness and into the light: Nebraska's experience with mental retardation.* Washington, DC: American Association on Mental Retardation.

Scheurich, J.J., & Skrla, L. (2003). *Leadership for equity and excellence.* Thousand Oaks, CA: Corwin.

Schon, D.A. (1983). *The reflective practitioner. How professionals think in action.* New York, NY: Basic Books.

Schraeder, T. (2013). *A guide to school services in speech-language pathology.* San Diego, CA: Plural Publishing.

Schwarz, P., & Kluth, P. (2008). *You're welcome: 30 innovative ideas for the inclusive classroom.* Portsmouth, NH: Heinemann.

Silberman, M. (1996). *Active learning: 101 strategies to teach any subject.* Boston, MA: Allyn & Bacon.

Snell, M., & Janney, R. (2005). *Teacher's guides to inclusive practices: Collaborative teaming* (2nd ed.). Baltimore, MD: Paul H. Brookes Publishing Co.

Snow, K. (2008). *To ensure inclusion, freedom, and respect for all, it's time to embrace people first language.* Retrieved from http://www.disabilityisnatural.com/explore/people-first-language

Stainback, S., & Stainback, W. (1996). *Inclusion: A guide for educators.* Baltimore, MD: Paul H. Brookes Publishing Co.

Strully, J.L., & Strully, C. (1996). Friendships as an educational goal: What we have learned and where we are headed. In S. Stainback & W. Stainback (Eds.), *Inclusion: A guide for educators* (pp. 141–154). Baltimore, MD: Paul H. Brookes Publishing Co.

Swinth, Y., Spencer, K.C., & Leslie, L. (2007). *Occupational therapy: Effective school-based practices within a policy context* (Center on Personnel Studies in Special Education No. OP-3). Retrieved from http://www.copsse.org

Tashie, C., Shapiro-Barnard, S., & Rossetti, Z. (2006). *Seeing the charade: What people need to do and undo to make friendships happen.* Nottingham, United Kingdom: Inclusive Solutions.

Taylor, R.L., Smiley, L.R., & Richards, S.B. (2009). *Exceptional students: Preparing teachers for the 21st century.* New York, NY: McGraw-Hill.

Theoharis, G. (2009). *The school leaders our children deserve: 7 keys to equity, social justice, and school reform.* New York, NY: Teachers College Press.

Thousand, J., Villa, R., & Nevin, A. (2007). *Differentiating instruction: Collaborative planning and teaching for universally designed learning.* Thousand Oaks, CA: Corwin.

Tomlinson, C.A. (2004). *How to differentiate instruction in the mixed ability classroom* (2nd ed.). Alexandria, VA: ASCD.

Topchik, G. (2001). *Managing workplace negativity.* New York, NY: AMACOM.

Turnbull, H.R., Turnbull, A.R., Shank, M., & Smith, S.J. (2004). *Exceptional lives: Special education in today's schools* (4th ed.). Upper Saddle River, NJ: Merrill/Prentice Hall.

Udvari-Solner, A. (1997). Inclusive education. In C.A. Grant & G. Ladson-Billings (Eds.), *Dictionary of multicultural education* (pp. 141–144). Phoenix, AZ: Oryx Press.

Udvari-Solner & Kluth. (2008). *Joyful learning: Active and collaborative learning in inclusive classrooms.* Thousand Oaks, CA: Corwin.

U.S. Department of Education. (2004). *Twenty-fourth annual report to Congress on the implementation of the Individuals with Disabilities Education Act.* Washington DC: Author.

U.S. Department of Education. (2007, September). *Twenty-seventh annual report to Congress on the implementation of the Individuals with Disabilities Education Act, 2005* (Vol. 1). Washington, DC: Author.

U.S. Department of Education, Office of Special Education Programs, Data Analysis System (DANS). (2011). OMB#1820-0043: *"Children with Disabilities Receiving Special Education Under Part B of the Individuals with Disabilities Education Act" 2011.* Washington, DC: Author. Retrieved from http://www.ideadata.org/

Villa, R.A., & Thousand, J.S. (Eds.). (2005). *Creating an inclusive school* (2nd ed.). Alexandria, VA: Association for Supervision and Curriculum Development.

Villa, R.A., Thousand, J.S., & Nevin, A.I. (2008). *A guide to co-teaching: Practical tips for facilitating learning* (2nd ed., pp. 169–171). Thousand Oaks, CA: Corwin Press.

Villa, R.A., Thousand, J.S., & Nevin, A.I. (2010). *Collaborating with students in instruction and decision making: The untapped resource.* Thousand Oaks, CA: Corwin.

Weil, S. (2001). *The need for roots.* London, United Kingdom: Routledge.

Wheatley, M.J. (2002). *Turning to one another: Simple conversation to restore hope in the future.* San Francisco, CA: Berrett-Koehler Press.

Will, M. (1986). *Educating students with learning problems: A shared responsibility.* Washington, DC: U.S. Department of Education, Office of Special Education and Rehabilitative Service.

Williams, R. (Presenter/Interviewer), & Thompson, S. (Interviewee). (2008, August 24). Hearing impairment: A personal story [Radio series episode]. In Seega, B. (Executive Producer), *Ockham's razor.* Sydney, Australia: ABC Radio National. Retrieved from http://www.abc.net.au/rn/ockhamsrazor/stories/2008/2342555.htm

Index

Page numbers followed by *b*, *f*, and *t* indicate boxes, figures, and tables, respectively.

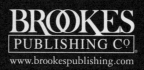
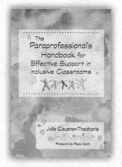
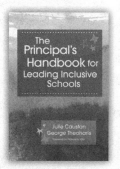
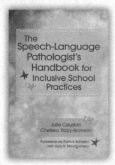
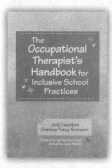